Antiviral Therapy

E. Blair[a], *G. Darby*[a], *G. Gough*[a], *E. Littler*[a],
D. Rowlands[b], *M. Tisdale*[a]

[a]Glaxo Wellcome Medicines Research Centre, Gunnels Wood Road,
Stevenage, SG1 2NY, UK

and

[b]Microbiology Department, University of Leeds, Leeds LS2 9JT, UK

ßIOS
SCIENTIFIC
PUBLISHERS

© BIOS Scientific Publishers Limited, 1998

First published 1998

A CIP catalogue record for this book is available from the British Library.

ISBN 1-85996-070-7

BIOS Scientific Publishers Ltd
9 Newtec Place, Magdalen Road, Oxford OX4 1RE, UK
Tel. +44 (0)1865 726286. Fax +44 (0)1865 246823
World Wide Web home page: http://www.Bookshop.co.uk/BIOS/

DISTRIBUTORS

Australia and New Zealand
  Blackwell Science Asia
  54 University Street
  Carlton, South Victoria 3053

India
  Viva Books Private Limited
  4325/3 Ansari Road, Daryaganj
  New Delhi 110002

Published in the United States of America, its dependent territories and Canada by Springer-Verlag New York Inc., 175 Fifth Avenue, New York, NY 10010-7858, in association with BIOS Scientific Publishers Ltd.

Published in Hong Kong, Taiwan, Singapore, Thailand, Cambodia, Korea, The Philippines, Indonesia, The People's Republic of China, Brunei, Laos, Malaysia, Macau and Vietnam by Springer-Verlag Singapore Pte. Ltd, 1 Tannery Road, Singapore 347719, in association with BIOS Scientific Publishers Ltd.

Production Editor Andrea Bosher.
Typeset by Banbury Pre-Press, Banbury, UK.
Printed by Biddles Ltd, Guildford, UK.

Contents

Abbreviations

3TC	3′-thiaribofuranonsyl-βL-cytosine (Epivir/lamivudine)
5FU	5-fluorouracil
AIDS	acquired immunodeficiency syndrome
araA	adenosine arabinose (vidarabine)
ACV	aciclovir
AZT	3′-azido-3′-deoxythymidine (zidovidine)
BPV	bovine papillomavirus
BVaraU	5-bromovinylarabinosyl uracil (sorivudine)
car	*cis* activation region
CDR	complementarity determining regions
CIN	cervical intraepithelial neoplasia (CIN1, CIN2, CIN3)
CNS	central nervous system
COPV	canine oral papillomavirus
CRPV	cottontail rabbit papillomavirus
crs	*cis*-repression sequence
CTL	cytotoxic T lymphocyte
d4T	2′,3′-didehydro-3′-deoxythymidine (stavudine)
DANA	2-deoxy-2,3-dehydro-*N*-acetyl neuramic acid
ddC	2′,3′-dideoxycytidine/(zalcitabine)
ddI	2′,3′-dideoxyinosine/(Didanosine)
dGTP	2′-deoxyguanosine-5′-triphosphate
DTH	delayed-type hypersensitivity
dTTP	2′-deoxythymidine triphosphate
eAg	e antigen (HBV)
EBV	Epstein–Barr virus
EIA	enzyme immunoassay
EV	epidermodysplasia verruciformis
FDC	follicular dendritic cells
FDG	2′-fluoro deoxyguanosine
FIAU	2′-deoxy-2′-fluoroarabinofuranosyl-5-iodouracil (fialuridine)
GM-CSF	granulocyte macrophage colony-stimulating factor
GST	glutathione-S-transferase
HA	hemagglutinin
HAV	hepatitis A virus
HBsAg	surface antigen protein of HBV

HBV	hepatitis B virus
HCV	hepatitis C virus
HDV	hepatitis delta virus
HEV	hepatitis E virus
HFV	human foamy virus
HGV	hepatitis G virus
HHV-6	human herpes virus-6
HHV-7	human herpes virus-7
HHV-8	human herpes virus-8
HIV	human immunodeficiency virus
HPV	human papillomavirus
HSV	herpes simplex virus
HTLV-1	human T-cell leukemia type 1
ICAM	intercellular adhesion molecule
IFN	interferon
IM	infectious mononucleosis
IN	integrase
INS	instability sequence
IRES	internal ribosome entry site
IUdR	5-Iodo-2´-deoxyuridine
IVIG	intravenous immuno-globulin
KS	Kaposis' sarcoma
LAMP1	lysosomal-associated membrane protein 1
LATs	latency associated transcripts
LCC	lymphocyte chemoattractant factor
LCR	long control region
LTR	long terminal repeat
mAb	monoclonal antibody
MHC	major histocompatability complex
NA	neuroaminidase
nef	negative factor
NNRTI	nonnucleoside RT inhibitor
NRE	negative response element
NSI	nonsyncytium inducing
ORF	open reading frame
PBMC	peripheral blood mononuclear cells
PCP	pneumocytosis carinii pneumonia
PCR	polymerase chain reaction
PIN	penile intraepithelial neoplasia
PMEA	(phosphonyl methoxy ethyl) adenine
PRI	HIV protease inhibitor
rIFN	recombinant interferons
RNaseH	ribonuclease H of HIV
RRE	rev response element
RSV	respiratory syncytial virus

RSaV	Rous sarcoma virus
RSVIG	RSV enriched immuno-globulin
RT	reverse transcriptase
RTI	HIV reverse transcriptase inhibitor
SAR	structure–activity relationship
SI	syncytium inducing
SIL	squamous intraepithelial lesions
SCC	squamous cell carcinoma
SU	surface
TK	thymidine kinase
TM	transmembrane
UTR	untranslated region
VLP	virus-like particles
WHO	World Health Organization

Preface

This has been a period of unsurpassed advances and challenges for the therapy of viral infections. It began with the discovery of a selective inhibitor of herpes viruses, aciclovir, which had a dramatic impact in the treatment and management of these diseases. However we were all unprepared for the appearance of two new viral diseases. HIV arrived with its enormous impact both for society and for the individuals and their families and friends. In the case of hepatitis C virus (HCV), its recognition revealed the alarming frequency of infection and long-term consequences. It is true to say that, as yet, the full impact of HCV on society has yet to be understood. The millennium finishes on a more hopeful note. Having recovered from the shock caused by the emergence of HIV and HCV, the scientific community, both academic and industrial, has provided insights into the nature of these diseases. We now have, after several years of unfulfilled hope, a cocktail of drugs which, although still not ideal, offer the prospect of long term supression of HIV. One effect of the emergence of HIV has been that it has provided a stimulus to discover novel types of inhibitors for other viral infections. Indeed new drugs are waiting in the wings to tackle more traditional, but none the less still important viral diseases, such as influenza, hepatitis B and respiratory syncytial virus. It is true, however, to say that we are only just at the beginning of being able to treat HCV.

This monograph will describe the history of development of antivirals and their current status. Each of the chapters on herpes viruses, hepatitis viruses, HIV, respiratory viruses and papilloma viruses also describe those agents which are about to enter the clinic in trials or be licensed for medical use. As with many areas of medicine, some of these agents will fail due to factors such as unexpected toxicity or lack of efficacy. Others will make it all the way and will become one of the battery of drugs for the clinician to use. An examination of recent drugs in development reveals that it is impossible to predict with any great confidence whether a given drug will be a breakthrough in therapy and which will be one of yesterdays false panaceas.

We conclude with a chapter which we openly admit is a collection of short essays on a variety of topics that failed to make it into the main chapters. These topics are too close to our scientific interests not to make the reader aware of them. Like the fledgling drugs described above, some of these essays may, in time, prove our insight while others may return to haunt us with their amazing inaccuracy!

Finally we would like to thank Allison Webster, Jane Crooks, Karen Biron and Todd Reinhart for their comments on various chapters and also thank Rob Young for providing electronic copies of the chemical structures shown in this monograph. Our special thanks goes to Caroline Yeldham for her sterling assistance in preparing the diagrams and manuscripts for submission to the publishers. Finally we would like to thank David Harper and BIOS for their help and patience in this protracted project.

Eddie Blair
Graham Darby
Gerald Gough
Eddy Littler
Dave Rowlands
Margaret Tisdale

Chapter 1

Development of antiviral chemotherapy

1.1 History: the origins of antiviral drug development

Viruses are responsible for many of the world's most serious diseases, and although they have been the focus of intensive research over the years they remain challenging organisms with which to work. Superficially they are the simplest of organisms with a relatively small complement of genes (anything between 5 and 200) and a very straightforward life-style. However, their replication is intracellular, and they make up for their genetic simplicity by a heavy reliance on the machinery of the host cell. Their intracellular site of replication and the intimate relationship they establish with the host cell make it extremely difficult to attack a virus infection without causing significant damage to the host organism. Furthermore, the viruses themselves are extraordinarily varied in their genetic organization and in the strategies they employ for their replication (*Figure 1.1*), and this in turn means that we must adopt different strategies in each case if we are to tackle them successfully. In this book we deal with viruses of major importance in human disease.

The main characteristics of the viruses covered are summarized in *Table 1.1*. This is by no means a comprehensive list of the viruses that are important in human disease, but it reflects those areas where antiviral chemotherapy is having, or is likely to have, significant impact.

When antiviral chemotherapy was in its infancy in the 1940s and 1950s, a major problem was the lack of convenient tissue culture systems in which the effects of potential drug molecules could be assessed. In those early years, before the development of tissue culture systems, viruses were generally grown in whole animals and this severely constrained the experimental work which could be done. Despite the severe difficulties, headway was made and a handful of molecules with antiviral properties was identified. The development of tissue culture in the mid-1950s, allowed many viruses to be grown and tested in well-controlled systems and provided a powerful stimulus to the whole area. Thus, considerable momentum built up through the 1960s and 1970s resulting in a number of molecules being tested in man and a few being registered for treatment of disease. However, it is in

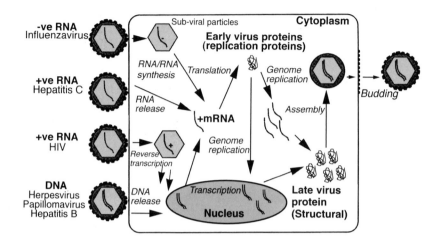

Figure 1.1: Virus replication strategies. Viruses enter cells through attachment to receptors on the cell surface. Once the cell is penetrated, subsequent events depend upon the nature of the virus genome. Positive-strand RNA genomes usually engage the cell's translation machinery, whereas DNA genomes usually penetrate the nucleus and are transcribed. With several viruses the initial events occur in virus-derived particles and are mediated by virus-coded particle enzymes. Thus, negative-strand RNA viruses contain a polymerase that synthesizes a positive-strand mRNA copy, and retroviruses contain reverse transcriptases that make DNA copies of the virus RNA genome. Similarly, the later events will also vary according to the virus but will usually involve replication of the virus genome, assembly of new particles and their release from the cell. In the case of retroviruses and hepatitis B, the amplification of the genome is driven by the transcription process rather than by newly synthesized virus-specific machinery.

the past decade that antiviral chemotherapy has 'come of age'. Most of this book deals with recent developments in the field, but in this introductory chapter an attempt is made to put these into a historical perspective.

1.2 Early antivirals

1.2.1 Thiosemicarbazones

Perhaps not surprisingly, the focus of antiviral research in the early years was diseases such as smallpox and poliomyelitis, which were considered major scourges of mankind. Indeed, the earliest antiviral molecules to be described, back in 1950, were the thiosemicarbazones, and they were active against smallpox virus, as well as other DNA viruses such as herpesviruses. The first antiviral to be tested extensively in man, isatin-β-thiosemicarbazone (methisazone), was a member of this class.

Table 1.1: Viruses of importance in human disease against which antiviral drugs are available

Family	Morphology	Genetic characteristics	Virus	Disease
Flaviviruses	Icosahedral enveloped	Positive-strand RNA Approximately seven genes	Hepatitis C	Chronic hepatitis, cirrhosis and liver cancer
Orthomyxoviruses	Filamentous enveloped	Negative-strand, segmented RNA eight genes	Influenza A and B	Respiratory infection with fever, myalgia and malaise
Retroviruses	Icosahedral enveloped	Positive-strand RNA 15 genes	Human immunodeficiency virus (HIV)	Acquired immune deficiency syndrome
Papillomaviruses	Icosahedral	Circular double-stranded DNA, 10 genes	Human papillomavirus	Genital warts
Herpesviruses	Icosahedral enveloped	Linear double-stranded DNA genome 70–150 genes	Herpes simplex virus	Cold sores and herpes genitalis
			Varicella-zoster virus	Chicken pox and shingles
			Cytomegalovirus	Cytomegalic inclusion disease (new-born) and retinitis (immunocompromised)
Hepadnaviruses	Icosahedral enveloped	Circular DNA genome (partially double-stranded) four genes	Hepatitis B virus	Chronic hepatitis, cirrhosis and liver cancer
Arenaviruses	Complex, enveloped	Ambisense RNA, four genes	Lassa fever	Hemorrhagic fever
Paramyxoviruses	Helical enveloped	Negative-strand RNA $\geq$ six genes	Respiratory syncytial virus	Bronchiolitis, pneumonia

Methisazone had been shown to be active against poxviruses using a model in which the virus was grown in the allantoic membrane of a fertile hen's egg. Subsequent work using a mouse model showed it to have efficacy *in vivo* against vaccinia virus (the smallpox vaccine strain). It was tested in the clinic in India in the early 1960s for the treatment of smallpox infection and for prophylaxis of individuals who had been exposed to the infection during an epidemic. Although these trials suggested some efficacy of the drug as a post-exposure prophylactic, disappointingly, there was little evidence for treatment efficacy. The drug was not developed further and the success of the World Health Organization (WHO) smallpox eradication campaign which was based on vaccination led to diminished interest in the poxviruses as drug targets.

It was another family of large DNA viruses, the herpesviruses, which were the first viruses to succumb to antivirals in the clinic.

1.3 The first nucleoside analogs

Although several other classes of molecule with antiviral activity were described in the early 1960s, only the nucleoside analogs have stood the test of time. Surprisingly, these molecules emerged initially, not from antiviral programs, but as a spin off from the search for anticancer drugs.

1.3.1 The pyrimidine deoxynucleoside analogs

5-Iodo-2′-deoxyuridine (IUdR) was one of many nucleoside analogs synthesized as a potential anticancer drug. The expected target of such molecules was the cellular DNA replication machinery, since they are analogs of the precursors of natural building blocks used in DNA synthesis, the deoxynucleoside triphosphates (*Figure 1.2*). However, just as cell division, and therefore cellular proliferation in tumors, depends on the replication of DNA, so DNA replication is the central event in the multiplication of DNA viruses, an infected cell producing many thousands of virus particles, each containing a newly synthesized DNA genome. It was therefore a logical extension of the work on anti-tumor compounds to test drugs in this class for efficacy against DNA viruses. The obvious targets at the time, because of their clear involvement in human disease, were herpesviruses and poxviruses.

It was soon shown that IUdR effectively blocks the replication of herpes simplex virus in culture and this was rapidly followed up with experiments in animal models which showed that the drug reduced the duration and severity of infection in the rabbit eye. These impressive results in animals were quickly translated into man and IUdR was registered for clinical use in herpes keratitis. It has remained in use to this day.

The development of IUdR was a success story but it also highlighted many of the potential pitfalls for antivirals. Although the molecule is a potent inhibitor of herpes simplex virus replication, unfortunately its activities are not restricted to the virus alone. They are also directed towards normal cells and this results in significant cytotoxicity. While this is not a serious problem if the drug is applied

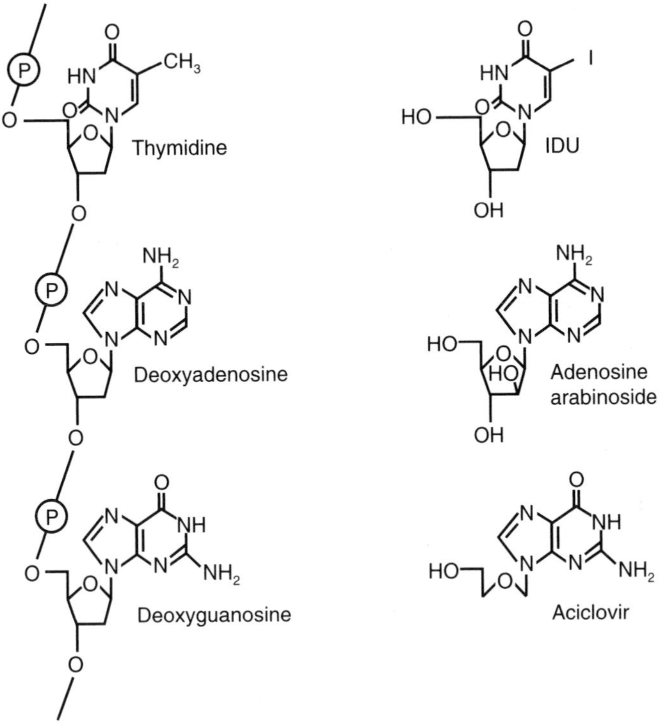

Figure 1.2: Antiherpes nucleoside analog. This figure shows the relationship between some of the nucleoside analogs and their natural counterparts. On the left is represented a hypothetical strand of DNA containing the natural nucleosides thymidine, deoxyadenosine and deoxyguanosine, and on the right are corresponding antiviral nucleoside analogs. Although the DNA strand is made up of nucleosides linked through monophosphate ester groups, the actual building blocks used are nucleoside 5′-triphosphates.

topically to external surfaces of the body, if it is administered systemically and gains access to internal organs the picture is quite different. In fact the cytotoxicity of the molecule results in a range of undesirable side-effects from alopecia (loss of hair), to more serious effects such as anemia and neutropenia, and in the long-term, carcinogenicity.

This illustrates one of the most important principals for antivirals. Since viruses are obligate intracellular parasites that depend on the cell for many of their replicative functions, many molecules which interfere with these cellular functions also block virus replication. However, such molecules are likely to have limited value as antiviral drugs because of their unwanted side-effects. The aim in developing antivirals must therefore be to develop molecules which selectively inhibit replication by hitting those gene products which are encoded by the virus and whose functions are absolutely necessary for replication. This goal was not to be achieved for at least another decade.

As well as being the first antiviral to be registered, it is also interesting to reflect that the discovery of IUdR had a relatively rational basis, being tested against DNA viruses because of its potential to inhibit DNA replication. This was at a time when virtually all other drugs in use had been discovered by serendipity or through random screening programs. Furthermore, the discovery of IUdR generated considerable interest in nucleoside analogs, and this class of molecule was to provide the life blood of antiviral research for many years to come.

In fact, the next generation of antivirals was heralded by the discovery of the antiherpes activity of a purine nucleoside analog, adenosine arabinoside (araA or vidarabine: see *Figure 1.2*).

1.3.2 Adenosine arabinoside

AraA was shown to be somewhat more selective than IUdR and to have efficacy in the treatment of serious, life-threatening herpes infections such as encephalitis and neonatal herpes. It represented the second landmark in the story of antivirals, as it was the first drug to be registered in the US for systemic use. However, there are two aspects of this drug which markedly reduce its utility. Firstly, in common with many nucleoside analogs, it has extremely poor oral bioavailability and so if systemic exposure is required the drug must be given intravenously. This, of course, ruled out the use of the drug for less serious infections where a convenient dosing regimen is an essential pre-requisite. Secondly, a more serious shortcoming of the molecule is its sensitivity to metabolism *in vivo*; the enzyme responsible, adenosine deaminase, cleaving the 6-amino group from the purine base, thereby considerably reducing the *in vivo* activity of the compound.

In order to tackle the second of these problems, attempts were made to develop inhibitors of adenosine deaminase. These, it was reasoned, might improve the efficacy of araA if given concurrently with the antiviral. The obvious starting point for potential inhibitors of adenosine deaminase was amongst analogs of the enzyme substrate and it was here that the search began. However, as so often happens in science, the path did not lead in the expected direction, but rather, to a far more important and unexpected prize.

1.4 The discovery of aciclovir

Among the molecules investigated as potential inhibitors of adenosine deaminase, were adenosine analogs with modified sugar moieties. In particular there was a series of analogs in which the sugar ring had been opened by removal of one or more carbon atoms. While investigating this series it was noticed that some members appeared to have antiviral activity in their own right. This observation prompted a far more thorough investigation which culminated in the discovery of 9-(2-hydroxyethoxymethyl)-guanine (aciclovir). This molecule was to set new standards for antivirals and was destined to become one of the world's most successful drugs (see *Figure 1.2*).

The first antiviral testing of aciclovir showed it to be extremely potent against herpes simplex virus (HSV) but not against any other family of viruses. Although its lack of activity against RNA viruses such as influenza and polio was not surprising, remarkably, it was also completely inactive against DNA viruses such as adenovirus and pox. Subsequently it was shown to have activity against other human herpesviruses such as varicella-zoster (VZV) and Epstein–Barr (EBV), although the activity was somewhat less than that against herpes simplex virus. It was also shown to be weakly active against human cytomegalovirus (HCMV). Aciclovir, therefore appears to be active against herpesviruses, but not against other families of viruses. However, over and above its antiviral profile, the most remarkable feature of aciclovir was its selectivity. Unlike all previous antivirals, which to a greater or lesser extent modulated normal cellular functions, aciclovir was essentially inert in uninfected cells. This selectivity, coupled with its potent activity against herpesviruses, was a major factor in insuring the success of this molecule in the clinic, where aciclovir was to become the treatment of choice for most herpesviral infections. In order to understand the selectivity of this molecule it is necessary to consider its mode of action.

The molecular target for aciclovir is the virus encoded DNA polymerase which is at the heart of the DNA replication machinery. This is an enzyme which is absolutely essential for virus multiplication, since without it there can be no replication of the viral genetic information. It is not the nucleoside analog itself which blocks the enzyme, but an activated form, the triphosphate, which mimics 2′-deoxyguanosine-5′-triphosphate (dGTP), one of the natural DNA building blocks. DNA polymerase mistakes aciclovir triphosphate for dGTP and incorporates it into the growing DNA chain. Because of its structure, specifically the lack of a 3′-carbon atom in the sugar, further elongation of the DNA chain is blocked. This mechanism of inhibition of DNA replication, which insures that the analog cannot be incorporated into mature DNA, is an important additional safety feature of the molecule. Incorporation of a nucleoside analog into mature cellular DNA, with its potential to induce mutations through replication errors, could have serious consequences.

The question that arises is why, if aciclovir triphosphate can have such a profound effect on DNA replication, is it not toxic to normal cells? The answer is that normal cells are not exposed to phosphorylated forms of the drug which would have the potential to interfere in purine nucleotide metabolism and/or DNA replication. Activation of the drug requires three kinase activities to be present in the cell. The first must be capable of converting aciclovir to its monophosphate, and it is this activity which is absent from the uninfected cell. In contrast, in the virus-infected cell an enzyme appears which is encoded by the virus genome and which is capable of phosphorylating aciclovir to its monophosphate. This enzyme, thymidine kinase, is normally responsible for phosphorylating thymidine to thymidine monophosphate, but it has the capability of recognizing a wide range of substrates for phosphorylation including the natural substrates thymidine monophosphate and the pyrimidine nucleoside, deoxycytidine. It is the broad substrate recognition properties of this enzyme which play right into the hands of the drug 'designer' (*Figure 1.3*).

Aciclovir was discovered in 1974, but it was during the 1980s that the full

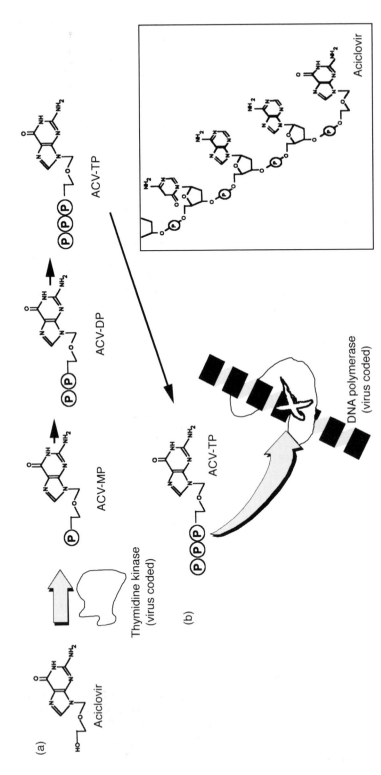

Figure 1.3: Mode of action of aciclovir. Although aciclovir itself is relatively inert in normal cells, in the infected cell it is phosphorylated by the virus-coded kinase to monophoshate. Activation continues by cell enzymes converting the monophosphate through to the triphosphate. The triphosphate is a substrate for the virus DNA polymerase and aciclovir monophosphate is incorporated into the viral DNA where it causes chain termination (see inset).

clinical potential of the drug was realized. Like its predecessor IUdR, it was first registered for use in herpes keratitis. However, its more important usage has been in serious herpes infections, especially infections in the immunocompromised. Although in the early years these were generally transplant recipients or cancer patients on cytotoxic drugs, more recently the drug has been widely used to control herpes infections in severely immunocompromised individuals infected with HIV. Because of the excellent safety profile of the drug, which became increasingly apparent over the years as experience was gained in many millions of treated patients, it is also possible to use it prophylactically in healthy individuals to suppress recurrent herpes infections. This is particularly useful in individuals with genital herpes infections who suffer frequent recrudescences of disease. Both frequency and severity can be dramatically reduced by prophylaxis.

The discovery and development of aciclovir once again provided a stimulus to the antiviral area and injected an air of optimism and expectation. More specifically it generated considerable interest in acyclic nucleosides, as other groups began prospecting in this attractive area. Disappointingly, there have been relatively few developments beyond aciclovir. However, two molecules with interesting antiviral properties are ganciclovir and penciclovir (*Figure 1.4*).

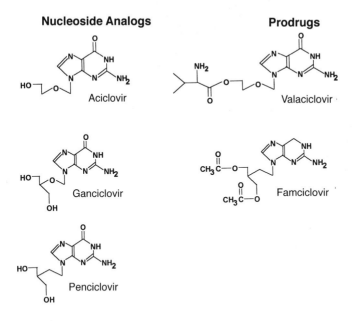

Figure 1.4: Acyclic nucleosides and prodrugs. Only three acyclic nucleosides have been registered for use against human disease to date, all against human herpesviruses. They all suffer from poor bioavailability and so prodrugs have been developed that deliver high drug concentrations when given orally. The prodrugs of aciclovir (valaciclovir) and penciclovir (famciclovir) are shown.

1.5 Ganciclovir and penciclovir

1.5.1 Ganciclovir

Ganciclovir is chemically a very close relative of aciclovir, having an additional carbon atom in the acyclic sugar moiety, equivalent to the 3′-carbon atom of the natural sugar (*Figure 1.4*). However, biologically, ganciclovir has quite distinctive properties, possessing good activity against human HCMV in addition to its activity against HSV and VZV. This additional antiviral activity is achieved at some cost, however, since ganciclovir is significantly less selective than aciclovir and its clinical use is therefore associated with significant side-effects, the most serious of which is bone marrow suppression. Because of this its use is limited to the treatment and control of life-threatening HCMV infections and to occasional use against herpes simplex variants resistant to aciclovir. An additional problem with this drug is its poor oral bioavailability and so it must be administered intravenously if systemic exposure is required.

More recently a valine ester ganciclovir prodrug (pro-ganciclovir) with improved oral bioavailability has been developed but the clinical results have so far been somewhat disappointing.

1.5.2 Penciclovir (and its prodrug, famciclovir)

Although chemically penciclovir appears to be closer to ganciclovir than aciclovir (*Figure 1.4*), its biological properties are more similar to those of aciclovir. Again, the bioavailability is poor and so an oral prodrug has been developed, the 6-deoxy diacetyl ester (famciclovir). To date clinical results suggest that in terms of efficacy against the herpesviruses this drug is not unlike aciclovir. Only experience will show whether or not it can match the excellent safety profile of aciclovir. One advantage is that the triphosphate of penciclovir has a long half-life in cells and so dosing can be less frequent than with aciclovir.

Finally, before leaving acyclic nucleosides, and remaining with the theme of prodrugs, a prodrug of aciclovir, valaciclovir, has also now been introduced.

1.6 Valaciclovir

The considerable clinical benefits of aciclovir have been achieved despite the relatively poor bioavailability of the drug (15–25%, depending on the dose administered). It was therefore reasoned that a prodrug approach might be useful with aciclovir if it could be achieved without prejudice to the excellent safety profile of the parent drug. The benefits to be expected from such an approach would be improved efficacy against the less sensitive viruses such as VZV or HCMV, and possibly a reduced dosing frequency.

The prodrug developed was the L-valyl-ester (*Figure 1.4*). This molecule has the advantage that when administered orally it is rapidly and completely broken down to aciclovir and the dietary amino acid, L-valine. The plasma levels of aciclovir achieved with the prodrug are 3–5 times the levels achieved with aciclovir itself, and this is now being translated into benefits in the clinic, both in terms of efficacy and more convenient dosing.

1.7 Further developments in pyrimidine nucleoside analogs

Although the acyclic nucleosides have stolen much of the limelight, work continued with 5-substituted pyrimidine nucleosides from the IUdR stable. However, experience here has been more sobering and has served to remind us of some of the potential hazards of working with nucleoside analogs. Two molecules taken recently into the clinic have unfortunately led directly or indirectly to serious consequences in a number of patients (*Figure 1.5*).

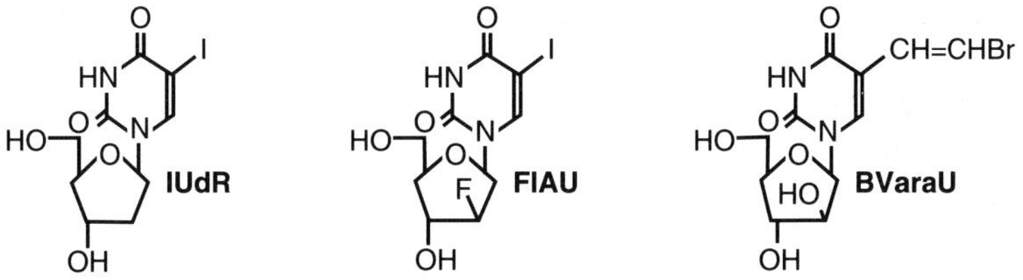

Figure 1.5: Further development of 5-substituted pyrimidines. FIAU (fialuridine) is closely related to IUdR, with the identical base and a modified sugar residue. BVaraU (or sorivudine) is less closely related with a modified 5-substituent on the base (the bromovinyl group) and also a modified sugar residue.

1.7.1 Sorivudine

Sorivudine (5-bromovinylarabinosyl uracil or BVaraU) is the most potent inhibitor of VZV so far discovered. It is also relatively selective, having little effect on uninfected cells. The drug was taken through clinical trials and was registered in Japan for the treatment of zoster (shingles). However, within a few months of the introduction of the drug into the market there were several deaths which were apparently drug related. Subsequent investigation revealed that the patients who died had all been treated concurrently with the 5-substituted pyrimidine analog, 5-fluorouracil (5FU), for underlying metastatic disease.

The problem related to the metabolism of these drugs *in vivo*. 5FU is a toxic drug, but the levels are effectively reduced by metabolism mediated by uracil reductase. Sorivudine, however, is metabolized by cleavage, and this releases the aglycone, 5-bromovinyluracil, which is also a potent inhibitor of uracil reductase. The net effect, therefore, is that uracil reductase inhibition results in elevated 5FU levels, which in turn may have lethal consequences in some people being treated simultaneously with both drugs. Such contraindications are an important consideration in situations where drug combinations are deliberate.

1.7.2 Fialuridine

Fialuridine (2´-fluoro-2´-deoxy-5-iodoarabinosyl uracil or FIAU) was originally synthesized many years ago, and major interest in the molecule was as a potential antiherpes drug. However, the introduction of aciclovir precluded its development for this purpose and interest in the molecule waned. More recently however, it was shown to have activity against hepatitis B virus, and so was taken into clinical trials to test its efficacy against chronic active hepatitis.

The initial safety evaluations in healthy and infected patients were encouraging and antiviral efficacy was seen. This prompted a Phase IIB trial in infected patients where the duration of treatment was increased significantly. It was during this trial that serious toxicity was encountered with several fatalities. The main target organs were the liver and pancreas and the effects appeared to be due a deterioration of mitochondrial function. Once it was realized that these effects were drug related the trials were terminated and development of the drug ceased.

These experiences provided a potent reminder that nucleoside analogs, with their potential to disrupt central functions of the cell, should be treated with great respect and we should not expect them all to have the safety profile of aciclovir. Despite this, nucleoside analogs have continued to have an important role in the control of virus diseases, the next area to receive considerable attention being that of HIV.

1.8 Nucleoside analogs for the treatment of HIV infection

With the realization in 1983 that AIDS was caused by a retrovirus, the hunt was on for effective antivirals to tackle this devastating disease. Perhaps not surprisingly, the first success was a nucleoside analog. Furthermore, this molecule, 3´-azido-3´-deoxythymidine (also known as AZT or zidovudine), had originally been synthesized almost 20 years earlier as a potential anticancer drug (*Figure 1.6*)

A feature of all retroviruses is that upon infection of a susceptible host cell the RNA genome of the virus is reverse transcribed into a double-stranded DNA copy. It is this process which is blocked by AZT which, like aciclovir, is incorporated into the growing DNA strand blocking any further chain elongation. However, a major difference between the mode of action of AZT and that of aciclovir is at the level of kinase activation. Whereas aciclovir is dependent on a virus-coded enzyme for activation, AZT is activated entirely by host cell enzymes. It is this non-specific activation process which leads to the markedly inferior selectivity of AZT compared with that of aciclovir.

In the clinic AZT was shown to be effective for the treatment of advanced HIV disease, although side-effects of the drug (primarily anemia and neutropenia) were quite severe in some individuals. Of even greater concern was that the benefits of treatment were not sustained, and after a year or two of treatment the patient's condition once again began to decline. It is now clear that the major reason for the loss of efficacy of the drug over time is the development of drug-resistant virus in treated individuals.

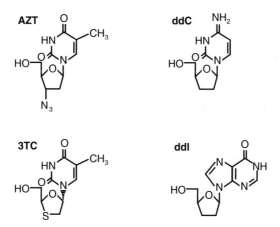

Figure 1.6: Dideoxynucleosides used in the treatment of HIV. AZT blocks DNA chain elongation because the 3´-position of the sugar lacks a hydroxyl group. Subsequent anti-HIV nucleosides such as ddC, 3CT and ddI exploit a similar mode of action.

The experience with AZT demonstrated clearly that drug treatment is an effective approach to the management of HIV infection, but it also highlighted the need to develop strategies to deal with drug resistance. The latter requires an armamentarium of alternative drugs which can be used in combination. Experience from the field of antimicrobials suggested that the best combinations would be those in which the component drugs each attacked a different molecular target, but the earliest available drugs after AZT were other dideoxynucleoside analogs targeted at reverse transcription and so these were the first to be assessed in com-bination therapy. 2´,3´-Dideoxycytidine (ddC) and 2´,3´-dideoxyinosine (ddI) were the first to be tried.

The first surprise was that virus which was highly resistant to AZT remained sensitive to both ddC and ddI. This dispelled one of the major fears concerning the use of drugs targeted at the same enzyme, that of cross-resistance. Furthermore, there was no interference between the drugs when used in combination and both appeared to provide additional benefit when used in combination with AZT. Another phenomenon was recognized early on from studies of patients who, after long periods of treatment with AZT, when the efficacy of AZT was declining, were switched to treatment with ddI. This was the phenomenon of resistance suppres-sion (*Figure 1.7*).

On switching to ddI therapy, some individuals whose virus had acquired resistance to AZT would, after a period of several months, begin to shed virus resistant to ddI but sensitive to AZT. It transpired that the virus retained the AZT resistance genotype but the mutation conferring resistance to ddI suppressed the

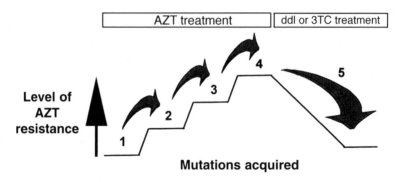

Figure 1.7: Suppression of AZT resistance. HIV in a patient treated with AZT acquires mutations in the *RT* gene which confer incremental resistance to AZT. Cessation of treatment with AZT and subsequent treatment with an alternative nucleoside such as ddI or 3TC may result in the acquisition of a further mutation conferring resistance to the second nucleoside, but suppressing the phenotypic effects of the AZT-induced lesions and causing reversion to AZT-sensitivity. See text for details.

AZT resistance phenotype. This observation suggested that there could be positive advantages in using two drugs which are targeted at the same molecule in combination. However, ddI is a relatively weak inhibitor of HIV and it was not until the far more potent drug, 3′-thiaribofuranosyl-βL-cytosine (3TC or epivir), was used in combination with AZT that the full potential of this phenomenon was revealed.

3TC is a very potent inhibitor of HIV but unfortunately, if used in monotherapy the efficacy of the drug is extremely short-lived as a single mutation in the reverse transcriptase gene reduces the sensitivity of the virus to the drug by about 1000-fold. However, this mutation behaves similarly to that described earlier which confers ddI resistance, suppressing resistance to AZT. When used in combination, the lesion conferring 3TC resistance appears rapidly but resistance to AZT is delayed, and the duration of benefit with the combination is considerably longer than with either drug alone.

Thus, there are now compelling reasons for looking at drugs aimed at the same molecular target. However, there could still be advantages in looking at different drug classes and the hunt for anti-HIV drugs did not end with the discovery of the dideoxynucleoside inhibitors of reverse transcriptase. The next important class of HIV drugs was also targeted at reverse transcriptase, albeit with a mechanism of action which is quite distinct.

1.9 Nonnucleoside inhibitors of HIV reverse transcriptase

Many groups set up screens to search for inhibitors of reverse transcriptase using the molecularly cloned HIV *RT* gene expressed in a heterologous system as the source of the enzyme. What was surprising was that almost every group which adopted this approach discovered potent inhibitors of the enzyme. What was even more surprising was that although these inhibitors represented many diverse classes of compound, their mode of action appeared to be the same. All were potent inhibitors of HIV-1 but not HIV-2 reverse transcriptases, and thus specific inhibitors of the HIV-1 virus. More recent structural work with enzyme/inhibitor complexes has shown that they bind to a common hydrophobic pocket adjacent to the active site of the enzyme and that this binding then distorts the relative positions of active site amino acid residues. It is presumably this distortion which results in the inactivation of the enzyme.

Unfortunately, the experience with these inhibitors in the clinic was similar to that with 3TC in that resistance rapidly developed and the efficacy of the drugs was short-lived. This resulted in a general lack of interest in these molecules until quite recently. It is now becoming apparent that successful control of HIV infection, perhaps not surprisingly, can only be achieved through the effective suppression of HIV replication. It is also clear that with effective suppression of virus replication with drug combinations, development of resistance can be considerably delayed. Drugs such as the nonnucleoside inhibitors of HIV may, therefore, because of their potency, have an important part to play in combinations in the future. Thus, although considerable emphasis was placed initially on how quickly a drug induced resistance, what is believed to be of greater importance now is the overall potency of drug combinations and the cross-resistance profiles of the individual components.

1.10 Protease inhibitors of HIV

The first successful inhibitors of HIV to exploit a different molecular target were the inhibitors of the aspartyl protease which is responsible for processing the gag–pol polypeptide precursor of both the structural *gag*-gene encoded proteins of the virus core and the *pol*-gene virus-specific replicative enzymes (the protease itself, reverse transcriptase and integrase). The development of drugs against this target relied on a rational approach (*Figure 1.8*) which began with knowledge of the protein cleavage sites recognized by the enzyme. This knowledge was used firstly to develop small peptide substrates of the enzyme and the peptide bond at the cleavage site was then modified to produce a non-cleavable inhibitor. Classical medicinal chemistry approaches were then employed to reduce both the molecular weight and the peptidic character of the inhibitors. By this route it was possible to develop highly potent and selective inhibitors of HIV.

The first of the protease inhibitors to be tested in the clinic was saquinavir. Despite its poor oral bioavailability it was found to be useful in combination with RT inhibitors. Subsequently other groups have been able to go even further using structural data on the interactions between inhibitors and the enzyme to develop a second generation of protease inhibitors, such as ritonavir and indinavir, with improved potency and bioavailabilty. These are now generating exciting results in the clinic although, not surprisingly, resistance to these molecules is emerging and their future use, as with RT inhibitors, will be in drug combinations.

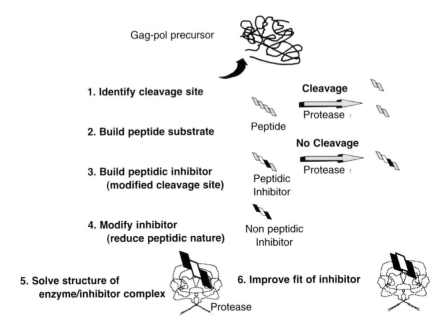

Gag-pol precursor

1. Identify cleavage site

Cleavage

Protease

2. Build peptide substrate

Peptide

No Cleavage

3. Build peptidic inhibitor
   (modified cleavage site)

Peptidic
Inhibitor

Protease

4. Modify inhibitor
   (reduce peptidic nature)

Non peptidic
Inhibitor

5. Solve structure of
   enzyme/inhibitor complex

Protease

6. Improve fit of inhibitor

Figure 1.8: Strategy for the development of protease inhibitors. First generation inhibitors (e.g. saquinavir) were developed using a biochemical approach based on knowledge of the specificity of the protease (steps 1–4). Later second generation inhibitors (e.g. ritonavir and indinavir) were developed further using structural data on enzyme/inhibitor complexes. Knowledge of the protease enzyme structure has also allowed the design of nonpeptidic inhibitors, for example XM323.

1.11 Other virus infections

Although the major achievements have been in the area of herpesviruses and HIV, there are many other virus infections which cause significant human disease, and several of these have received significant attention over the years.

1.11.1 Influenza virus infection

Influenza epidemics have had devastating effects on human populations. The natural variation of the virus ensures that immunity is relatively short-lived, and this variation leads to annual epidemics of disease, with the young and old being especially vulnerable. This makes influenza an attractive target for a therapeutic approach. In fact, one of the earliest antivirals to be discovered, amantadine, is an influenza virus-specific drug.

Amantadine. Amantadine and related molecules have been the subject of intensive research over the years, but it was not until quite recently that their mode of action was deduced. It became clear in the early studies that amantadine blocks an early event in the virus replication cycle. However, it was not until resistant viruses were obtained and the genetic loci of their lesions were mapped that it became clear that the target for these drugs is a small virus-coded protein termed M2. This focused attention on the function of the M2 protein which turned out to be totally novel for a virus-coded protein. It is now clear that the M2 protein aggregates in membranes to form an ion channel and it is believed that this channel regulates the pH of vesicles containing the virus. This is important for influenza virus because one of its major surface glycoproteins, hemagglutinin (HA), is sensitive to pH and undergoes a conformational change at low pH exposing a hydrophobic domain that promotes membrane fusion and virus entry into the cell. The M2 pump ensures that the pH is closely regulated so that this conformational change does not occur at an inappropriate time.

Although drug resistance allowed the mode of action of the drug to be worked out and opened up new and exciting avenues of research, it has proved a serious limitation with this drug. Almost all treated individuals shed resistant virus after a few days, and so anyone infected by these individuals is likely to be refractory to treatment.

Zanamivir. Although for many years amantadine and its analogs represented the only antiviral approach to influenza therapy, there are now some exciting alternatives appearing.

Apart from the hemagglutinin, on the surface of the influenza virus particle there is a second glycoprotein, the neuraminidase (NA). This is a surface enzyme which is able to remove the receptors recognized by hemagglutinin on the cell membrane and which is most probably involved in the escape of new virus particles from the cell. With information on the structure of the neuraminidase and its substrate it has been possible to design potent inhibitors of this enzyme. The first of these, zanamavir, is effective in animal models of disease (the mouse and the ferret), and currently being evaluated in the clinic.

1.11.2 Chronic viral hepatitis

Chronic viral hepatitis afflicts several hundred million people world-wide and many go on to develop severe liver disease such as cirrhosis or liver cancer. There are two viruses that are responsible for the majority of this disease, hepatitis B and hepatitis C, and they are the focus of considerable effort in the antiviral field. They are both difficult viruses, since neither replicates well in culture or in any convenient animal model. Nevertheless, there has already been some success in developing antivirals against hepatitis B virus (HBV).

Hepatitis B. Interferons have been used in the treatment of chronic active hepatitis caused by hepatitis B virus. The treatment is inconvenient and may be unpleasant for the patient because of the 'flu-like' symptoms that are a side-effect of interferon, but there is a proportion of patients who respond well and clear the infection.

With the more traditional small molecule antiviral agents, there was relatively little success until recently and, interestingly, it is spin-offs from other areas that have provided the excitement.

The antiherpes drug, famciclovir, has been shown to have activity against hepatitis B virus both in culture and in chronically infected patients. This result is surprising since it was believed that activation of this drug, like aciclovir, required the herpes-specific thymidine kinase. The implication is that, at least in the liver, there are host cell enzymes that can perform the initial phosphorylation step.

The second drug which has been shown to have activity against hepatitis B is the anti-HIV drug, 3TC. This is less surprising, since hepatitis B, like HIV, depends on reverse transcription by a virus-coded polymerase for its replication (see *Figure 1.9*).

What is surprising at first sight is that the rapid development of resistance seen with HIV does not appear to occur with HBV. One possible explanation lies in the compact arrangement of the hepatitis B genome which results in some overlap of coding regions from different genes. The putative active site of the polymerase is one such region and this may constrain the mutations allowed in this region. Whatever the explanation, in many patients this drug has been shown to have a profound and sustained effect on virus replication.

Hepatitis C. This virus, which is related to the flavi and pestiviruses was only discovered recently but nevertheless it is known to be responsible for liver disease in many millions of people throughout the world. As with hepatitis B there is some response to interferon treatment, although the infection recurs in most patients. So far there are no candidate antivirals for the treatment of this infection.

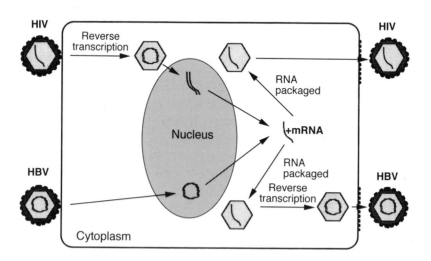

Figure 1.9: Dependence of HIV and hepatitis B on reverse transcription. Both HIV and hepatitis B have a reverse transcription step in their replication cycle. In the case of HIV, genomic RNA is reverse transcribed prior to integration into the chromosome of the cell, whereas in the case of hepatitis B, packaged RNA is reverse transcribed to make genomic DNA prior to particle release.

1.11.3 Papillomavirus

This is another virus which is particularly challenging because of its failure to grow in tissue culture systems. It is responsible for genital warts and infection with some variants predispose women to the development of cervical cancer, and it is therefore a worthwhile target for antivirals. Since the live virus cannot be used to search for potential drugs, an alternative approach is to search for inhibitors using screens against specific virus functions. Here again this virus is especially frustrating since it has a very small number of genes, and only one of them has so far been shown to have enzymatic activity, the *E1* helicase. As yet there are no strong candidate antivirals for this virus.

1.11.4 Lassa fever

Ribavirin, a somewhat unselective drug used largely for the treatment of respiratory syncytial virus infections in babies (see Chapter 4), is also active clinically against lassa fever, a severe hemorrhagic disease. The mechanism of action against lassa fever virus, an arenavirus, is unknown, but because of the severity of disease, it may be used in such cases.

1.12 Summary

In this introductory chapter the development of antivirals has been traced using examples from many different viruses. In the 1960s, IUdR demonstrated for the first time that it was possible to modulate a human viral infection using an antiviral drug but at the same time highlighted the need to develop selective agents. Twenty years later aciclovir established once and for all that it is possible to develop such selective drugs and that selectivity could be expected to correlate with an impressive safety profile. The lesson learned with HIV was that in treating chronic virus infections with long-term exposure to drugs, resistance is likely to become an issue. However, another important lesson is that resistance can be minimized with appropriate drug combinations, and not necessarily combinations of drugs from different classes.

All of these issues will be revisited in greater detail in later chapters and hopefully this should provide a comprehensive view of both the remarkable achievements so far and also the immense challenges ahead in this fast moving and exciting field. Whatever the future holds, the time when virus infections were considered untreatable are now behind us and we can confidently look forward to dramatic developments over the next few years.

Chapter 2

Chemotherapy of herpesvirus infections

2.1 Introduction: what is a herpesvirus?

The presence of herpesvirus-like particles has been reported from almost all eukaryotic organisms, including fungi. However, outside of those that infect mammals most of these viruses are relatively poorly characterized.

Traditionally the definition of what constitutes a herpesvirus is based upon the morphology of the virus particle and the observation that the members of the herpesvirus family have a double-stranded DNA genome which replicates in the nuclei of infected cells. Indeed it is reassuring that there has been good general agreement with the members of the herpesvirus family and its subdivisions based upon traditional characteristics and those based upon more recent molecular biological techniques.

2.1.1 Morphology

Examination of a herpesvirus under the electron microscope shows that it has an icosahedral nucleocapsid, approximately 100–110 nm in diameter, composed of 162 subunits (capsomeres). The nucleocapsid is surrounded by a membranous envelope which, although derived from the host cell also contains so-called spikes made up of a number of virus-coded glycoproteins. Between the nucleocapsid and the envelope there is an amorphous layer of proteins (largely virus coded) termed the tegument which is of indeterminate function although it is known to contain many of the proteins that initiate virus replication. The whole virion is approximately 120–300 nm in diameter. The significance, if any, of the size variation is unknown, indeed these differences are often resolved by the use of cryo electron microscopy, which preserves original structures more fully.

2.1.2 Genome

The herpesvirus genome is a linear double-stranded DNA molecule varying in length between approximately 80 and 220 kbp. The base composition (the percentage GC vs. AT) varies from 32 to 75%. This is amazing when one considers that the whole of the chordate genus does not vary beyond 40–44% GC. Genetic analysis shows that it is common for the herpesvirus genome to have 'domains' which contain unique sequences coding for viral genes surrounded by DNA sequences which are repetitive in nature (*Figure 2.1*).

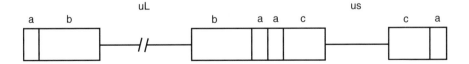

Figure 2.1: Genetic arrangement of herpes simplex virus genome. The herpes simplex virus genome consists of two genetically unique (u) regions (large L and small s), surrounded by repeat structures (labeled a, b and c). Other herpesviruses have similar repeat structures.

DNA sequence analysis has shown that there is considerable variation in the DNA sequence between different herpesviruses. However, the organization of the genome and the amino acid sequence of the encoded proteins demonstrate that they are genetically related. Some gene functions are shared by all members of the group (i.e. DNA polymerase, glycoproteins B and H, helicase, protease). Others are found only in one or maybe two members of the group (e.g. thymidylate synthetase or the EBV EBNA gene products).

Herpesvirus genes and their products can also be divided into those coding for 'early' virus events in the replication cycle (transcription and DNA replication) and those involved in 'late' events (such as virus assembly) and the viral structural components themselves. The virus 'early' genes are important clinically as they are the targets for current established antiviral chemotherapy (DNA polymerase). Similarly the late genes code for proteins (e.g. glycoproteins) which are the current choice for candidate sub-unit vaccines.

2.1.3 Replication and general biology

The typical replication cycle of a herpesvirus may be broken down into a number of stages. (1) Virus attaches and fuses to the cell surface. In the case of herpes simplex virus (HSV) this interaction is at least in part with heparin sulphate proteoglycan on the cell surface. Examples of cell receptors for other herpesviruses include the C3d receptor for Epstein–Barr virus (EBV). (2) Virus penetrates the cell membrane and uncoats, moving to the nucleus. (3) The virus particle contains a number of proteins which modify the host transcriptional apparatus making it more amenable to virus gene expression. (4) Virus transcription begins in a tem-

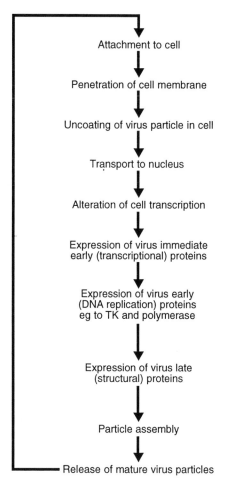

Figure 2.2: Typical life cycle of a herpesvirus.

porally coordinated manner, the first genes also being involved in modifying the host transcription apparatus, the second involved in the replication of the virus genome and the final phase being involved in virus particle formation and morphogenesis. In reality this three phase gene expression is an over-simplification with very few virus genes falling truly into any one class and most being found expressed (at varying amounts) throughout the whole virus life cycle. In the case of HSV the whole replication cycle is complete within 24 h (see *Figure 2.2*).

2.1.4 Latency

One important feature of the herpesviruses is that they have the ability to persist in a state that avoids the host immune response. This persistent state is known as latency and is lifelong. There are differences in the exact site of persistence of individual herpesviruses and hence the molecular mechanism by which latency is

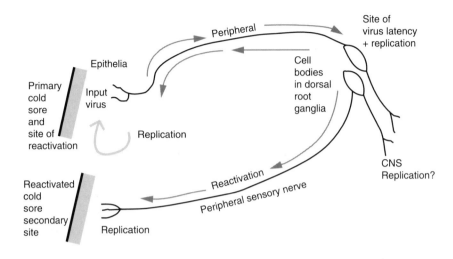

Figure 2.3: Infection and establishment of latency in HSV.

established and maintained. The ability of herpesviruses to form latent infections has enormous clinical implications that will be referred to in the rest of this chapter (see *Figure 2.3*).

2.1.5 Diseases caused by herpesviruses in humans

There are eight identified human herpesviruses, however only six have been studied in detail. The herpesviruses are the cause of many common infections in humans (*Table 2.1*). The patterns for the interaction of a herpesvirus and its host are very similar. After transmission [which is either by body fluids—HSV and EBV or respiratory—varicella-zoster virus (VZV)] the viruses cause a primary overt disease which is systemic in nature but is observed as being commonly of the skin. During this primary infection the viruses establish a latent infection in a specific cell type (for example neurones for HSV or B cells for EBV). There then follows a period of time, which may, in some cases be years, during which time the viruses are latent with no apparent adverse effect on their host. Finally due to a change in the environment of the host (immune status or a stimulus such as physical trauma) the herpesviruses reactivate causing a secondary infection, which may be singular as in the case of shingles or multiple as in the case of cold sores.

2.2 Herpes simplex virus

The first scientific description of HSV was in 1919 when Lowenstein reported the infectious nature of the disease. Some 10 years later a crucial observation was made that recurrences of herpes labialis occurred in patients who had previously

Table 2.1: Human herpesviruses

Virus	Primary disease	Recurrent disease	Site of latency	Other pathologies
HSV-1	Gingivitis	Cold sores	Neuronal	CNS (encephalitis)
HSV-2	Genital herpes	Genital herpes	Neuronal	CNS
VZV	Chickenpox	Shingles	Neuronal/ satellite cells	Visceral infection
HCMV	Cytomegalic disease in neonates. IM-like illness in adults	Eye, lung, gastrointestinal tract	Monocyte?	Serious disease only in immunocompromised and neonates
EBV	Infectious mononucleosis (IM)		B cell	Tumors B cell Hodgkin's and epithelial
HHV-6	Exanthum subitum		T cell?	
HHV-7	Exanthum subitum		?	Virus isolated from AIDS patients
HHV-8			?	Link to Kaposis' sarcoma and other malignancies

existing antibodies to the disease. This paradox remained until the ability of the virus to establish a latent infection and its consequence on disease pathology was understood. Herpes labialis is reported to occur in approximately 50% of the world's population and there are thought to be half a million primary cases of genital herpes infections each year in the USA alone.

Work by Nahmias *et al.* showed that there were two antigenically related but distinct viruses associated with oro-facial herpes (cold sores) and genital herpes (HSV-1 and 2 respectively). This antigenic difference is also reflected in genetic and DNA sequence variation. The 'above the belt, below the belt' distinction between HSV-1 and -2 has blurred since the 1960s albeit more so in some countries than others (Japan and UK have more HSV-1 genital disease than USA). HSV has been found world-wide. There are no animal vectors and no seasonal variation in transmission. Primary infection by HSV-1 has usually occurred by 5 years of age (this is heavily influenced by factors such as geography and socio-economic class) and is associated with gingivostomatitis or a febrile-type illness with pharyngitis. HSV-2 infections are generally spread by sexual contact and hence are rarely seen before the age of sexual maturity. While HSV-1 can also cause genital infections they are usually less severe and less prone to return. It is estimated that there are between 40–60 million people infected with HSV-2 in the USA alone.

Apart from the cold sores, primary infection by HSV can also establish a CNS infection in rare cases causing significant damage, morbidity and possibly death from encephalitis.

HSV is spread by close intimate contact between an infected individual and a naïve one, in that excreted virus must come into contact with a mucosal surface before it is inactivated by physical factors such as heat or dehydration. Virus replicates at the site of infection causing a small (perhaps at this stage imperceptible) rash. Next this virus infects local neurones and is transported to the dorsal root ganglia (trigeminal for HSV-1 and sacral for HSV-2) where it becomes latent. Experiments have shown that prior replication of the virus in the host is not essential to establish a latent infection. However, most authorities would agree that virus replication amplifies the resident pool making it a more efficient process. The virus may lie dormant in the ganglia for a period of time measured within weeks to years. At some point a stimulus such as immunosuppressive therapy, hormonal changes, physical or emotional trauma may trigger it to replicate. At this time the virus gives rise to oro-facial cold sores or genital sores depending upon the site of initial infection and hence the location of the dorsal root ganglia at which the virus has established latency.

2.2.1 HSV latency

Examination of latently infected ganglia from experimentally infected animals shows that, although some specific RNA transcripts are expressed, no protein products have been detected. Indeed detailed analysis of these latency associated transcripts (LATS) show that for some strains of HSV there is no significant open reading frame capable of being expressed as protein. The role of the LATS in herpesvirus latency is not clear, indeed some of the LATS identified for some animal herpesviruses clearly have a different mechanism of action than those of HSV.

Despite the fact that we do not understand the molecular basis of herpesvirus latency we are all too aware of its clinical consequences. In the 'normal' immune competent individual this may lead to several episodes of oro-facial cold sores or genital sores each year. Apart from the pain and discomfort that arises from such a reactivation there are other major implications in an individual's quality of life. Many people with genital herpes live in fear of infecting a partner (or a child during delivery through an infected birth canal). There is also the stigma of having a sexually transmitted disease. However, the consequences of latent herpesvirus infections for the immune compromised are potentially much more severe. Due to the ubiquitous nature of HSV there is a very high chance that an

HIV-infected individual or one undergoing transplantation will have a latent infection. Free from immune surveillance the latent HSV may reactivate to cause overt disease. In this case, however, as there is no limitation by the host immune response, the lesions rather than self-resolving may extend to form much more wide spread and persistent sores. Left untreated the virus may spread to internal organs such as the lung, leading to a potentially life-threatening condition.

Finally HSV is an important pathogen of the fetus and the new-born with some 1 in 3–5000 neonates in the USA being infected with HSV. The prognosis for such infections is variable, infection may be severe and disseminated, or localized infections of the skin or eye which respond well to standard antiviral therapy.

2.3 Varicella-zoster virus

Infection with VZV occurs apparently via the respiratory route (presumably via aerosols from an infected individual) although this model has not been confirmed. After infection of the mucous membranes there follows a viremia which distributes the virus to organs such as the liver and, via a secondary viremia, the virus then spreads to cutaneous epithelial cells. This results in the appearance of rash typical of chickenpox and an elevated temperature. A second target organ for VZV appears to be the lung cells (presumably VZV replicates here to release virus for subsequent infection) which can lead to one of the most serious complications of VZV namely pneumonia which has a high mortality rate (particularly in smokers). VZV also has a CNS involvement in its pathology with reports of encephalitis. Infection of the fetus is rare but serious. Whilst in childhood chickenpox can arguably be considered not to be a serious illness — the same cannot be said of the disease in adolescence and adulthood. In these cases a significant number of individuals develop infections of the lung which if not diagnosed early can have serious consequences, including death. Indeed there is considerable support for the use of antiviral therapy in all patients developing primary chickenpox outside of childhood.

During primary infection VZV establishes latency in the dorsal root ganglia where it remains dormant usually until middle to late age. There is some controversy as to whether the virus is latent in neuronal cells or in their associated satellite cells. There are no obvious homologs of the HSV LAT transcripts.

In some of VZV-infected people there will be no further reactivations. However, in those that do undergo reactivations, the result is the painful disease, shingles (zoster). Often the first symptoms of the onset of shingles is a prodome consisting of a feeling of malaise with fever and pain on, for example, the lower torso which after a few days becomes associated with a rash. The malaise will persist for a few days after the rash appears. The disease will normally progress for a period of 7–10 days during which time the vesicles will scab and heal and the associated pain will disappear. However, some cases do not follow this usual pattern. In these cases, whilst the lesions will heal, the pain will persist for a number of weeks or months. In extreme cases persistence can be for years. Risk factors for the likelihood of severe persistent symptoms include severity of pain before onset of rash (or early after rash has formed), age of patient and whether the patient is depressed. It is likely that prodomal pain or severe rash is an indicator of severe nerve damage and increases the risk of acute and or chronic pain. It is quite clear that antiviral intervention can have a positive impact on length and severity of pain and lesion healing if given early after onset of disease. However, once established the persistent pain itself is not amenable to antiviral therapy and treatment options include capsacin, sympathetic nerve blocks or physical barriers from clothing, chaffing is often a trigger factor for pain. However it is important to note that once established chronic pain in zoster is notoriously difficult to treat effectively and the treatments described above (capsacin etc) are used largely in desparation.

As in the case of HSV the ability of VZV to establish a latent infection in the majority of people makes it an important opportunistic infection in the immunocompromised. Most importantly, primary VZV infection (chickenpox) in the immunocompromised can lead to serious complications. For example VZV pneumonia in bone marrow or renal transplant recipients carries a high mortality.

2.4 Human cytomegalovirus

Human cytomegalovirus (HCMV) is highly species specific and is an important pathogen of the immune compromised, whilst only rarely causing recognizable clinical features in the immune competent individual. Natural transmission occurs by direct person-to-person contact or via common contacts. Virus has been identified in many if not all human secretions including breast milk, feces, urine and blood. Primary infection is not usually clearly identifiable and an immunologically normal individual may be found to periodically shed virus. Approximately 0.2–2% of new-borns in the USA are infected and this rate rapidly increases over the first 6 months of life. Other modes of transmission include sexual intercourse and via contaminated blood products.

True primary infection in the normal host is accompanied by little overt disease, although a mononucleosis-like illness is sometimes reported. Early during primary infection virus may be detected in epithelium of the oral cavity and this is followed by viremia. Other commonly infected organs include the kidney and the gastrointestinal system. Infections *in utero* have a high morbidity (including hearing loss and neurodevelopmental delay) and mortality. There are estimates that suggest that HCMV is the second most common cause of learning difficulties after Downs syndrome. The rate of transmission of HCMV from mother to fetus varies according to the immune status of the mother.

The infection of the immunocompromised by HCMV is of increasing importance. It is important to realize that the pattern of disease in organ transplant patients is different from that observed in HIV-infected people (indeed there is some variation within different types of organ transplant patients according to the severity of the immune suppressive therapy). In organ transplant patients, HCMV infection is associated with the development of pneumonitis. In HIV patients there is no general trend for HCMV to cause pneumonitis but instead it is associated with retinitis, with infections also in the gastrointestinal system and CNS. In all of these HCMV diseases, the mechanism of disease is not clear. In the case of pneumonitis there is evidence that in the latter established stages of the disease the driving mechanism is the immune response to HCMV and not primary virus replication and cytolysis.

The site at which HCMV establishes latency is not clear. Virus can be found at a number of sites including kidney and in monocytes The moncyte is thought to be a site of latency in the normal individual although the mechanism of maintenance of latency and the virus genes involved in the process are not known.

As described below, antiviral therapy of HCMV infections is far from satisfactory and often conflicts with anti-retroviral therapy used in HIV-infected individuals.

2.5 Epstein–Barr virus

Epstein–Barr virus was first identified in 1964 originating from a tumor biopsy from an African Burkitt's lymphoma patient. Indeed there is a strong correlation with prior EBV infection and endemic Burkitt's lymphoma. One of the most striking properties of EBV is its ability to transform B lymphocytes to form a permanent B-cell line. This *in vitro* capability and clinical observation have demonstrated an association of EBV with a number of human tumors including Burkitt's lymphoma, nasopharyngeal carcinoma, Hodgkin's disease and B-cell lymphomas of the immune compromised. Primary infection with EBV is via saliva, usually occurs in early childhood and is not usually associated with overt disease. Primary infection occurs in epithelial cells of the throat, although the virus may need to be amplified in B cells. After the host mounts an immune response, the virus replication is controlled but is thought to be incompletely repressed with continual chronic shedding of virus into the saliva occurring throughout life.

If infection is delayed until adolescence the individual may develop infectious mononucleosis (IM), also called glandular fever. This self-limiting disease is characterized by symptoms such as headache, pharyngitis and transient fever with associated lymphadenopathy, malaise and lethargy. Clinically, IM is not considered by many (rightly or wrongly) as requiring therapy. There is some evidence that suggests that the symptoms of IM are largely due to the immune response to EBV and that by the time a patient presents it is too late for antiviral therapy. However there have been only a few clinical trials that used agents such as aciclovir to test this hypothesis. Indeed a number of individuals can maintain symptoms of IM for a number of months or years and prevention of this possibility definately warrants consideration.

After primary infection EBV forms a latent infection in a B cell where it undergoes periodic asymptomatic reactivations resulting in virus in the saliva. The mechanism by which EBV establishes and maintains latency is well understood and, as might be expected due to the very different nature of the cell type, has little in common with the other herpesviruses.

In the immunocompromised reactivation can lead to B-cell lymphomas which are a common cause of death. However, in the case of the EBV-associated tumors, a latent or limited expression of the virus genome occurs, thus severely limiting the efficacy of antiviral therapy. Recent attempts at stimulating the hosts cytotoxic T-cell response in patients with EBV-associated tumors have been reported to show promise. In HIV patients, EBV has been shown to be the cause of oral hairy leukoplakia, a lesion on the tongue which is packed with virus particles. These lesions respond well to aciclovir therapy.

2.6 Human herpes virus-6

This virus was first isolated from a T-cell line established from an AIDS patient. It was soon discovered that over 90% of all populations are infected with HHV-6. The virus was subsequently shown to cause exanthem subitum (also known as roseola infantum), a common childhood disease with symptoms such as elevated temperature (>39°C) followed by a transient rash. More importantly HHV-6 has been shown to be neurotropic and associated with CNS disease in children, including convulsions, which may be repeated. The virus can be shown to be prevalent in the immune compromised where it may be associated with graft suppression/rejection.

The site of latency of HHV-6 is not established and neither is any clear relationship of disease due to reactivating virus. In addition this virus is closely related to HCMV and appears to be similar in the difficulty in treatment of disease.

2.7 Human herpes virus-7

A somewhat mysterious virus found in T cells with little apparent disease associations except exanthum subitum. Indeed in some patients it has been shown that infection by HHV-7 was beneficial for the disease outcome of HIV infection.

2.8 Human herpes virus-8

Originally identified by molecular analysis of a Kaposis' sarcoma (KS) biopsy this virus is now considered to be a possible causative agent in KS. Genetically closely related to EBV and some of the malignant primate herpesviruses, the mechanism by which it may cause KS is unclear but is seems as if virus replication is not required. Recent reports show that HHV-8 codes for a classical seven transmembrane protein capable of acting as a cytokine responsive oncogene, and a potential transforming oncogene has also been identified.

2.9 History of antiviral therapy

In the 1960s a number of nucleoside analogs such as 5-iododeoxyuridine had been developed for treatment of herpesvirus infections. However, the early drugs were metabolically unstable and toxic, preventing their use as systemic agents.

Modification of the nucleoside sugar as with adenosine arabinoside, led to improvements in stability but did not completely resolve these problems. The unsuitability of these nucleoside analogs is partially due to their deamination by the enzyme adenosine deaminase. In an attempt to reduce this deamination a number of nucleoside analogs were synthesized as potential adenosine deaminase inhibitors. In 1978 the nucleoside analog 9-(2-hydroxymethyl) guanine was reported by scientists at the Wellcome Foundation. As part of a routine program this compound was assessed in antiviral assays and was found to have its own intrinsic anti-herpesvirus activity. This discovery opened the era of modern antivirals and led to the awarding of the Nobel prize to the scientists who first synthesized and subsequently developed the antiviral — aciclovir (marketed as Zovirax™).

Information from the laboratory and from the clinic has shown that aciclovir is effective both prophylactically and therapeutically against HSV-1 and-2, VZV and for prophylaxis of HCMV. Given intravenously aciclovir is effective in suppressing HCMV and would be expected to show improved activity against HSV and VZV.

2.9.1 Mode of action of aciclovir

The structure of aciclovir is shown in *Figure 2.4*. It is not a true nucleoside, lacking a true cyclic sugar moiety. The mechanism by which aciclovir inhibits herpesvirus replication, as shown in *Figure 2.5*, has been elucidated by a variety of genetic and biochemical experiments and may be summarized as follows. Phosphorylation of the nucleoside by the virus-encoded thymidine kinase to its monophosphate, and synthesis of the di- and triphosphates by host cell kinases. It is the aciclovir triphosphate which is the antiviral agent, thus the drug itself could be considered a prodrug of the final active form. The triphosphate is recognized by the viral DNA polymerase and is incorporated into the replicating viral genome. Once inserted into the DNA, aciclovir, which lacks a 3′-hydroxyl group, causes a termination in DNA synthesis; this is termed obligate chain termination. This mechanism of obligate chain termination is thought by many to be one of the features of aciclovir that is important to its efficacy and perhaps more importantly, overall safety in the clinic. For example it will prevent cells being generated containing an aciclovir nucleoside substitution which, if it was to occur, could be mutagenic.

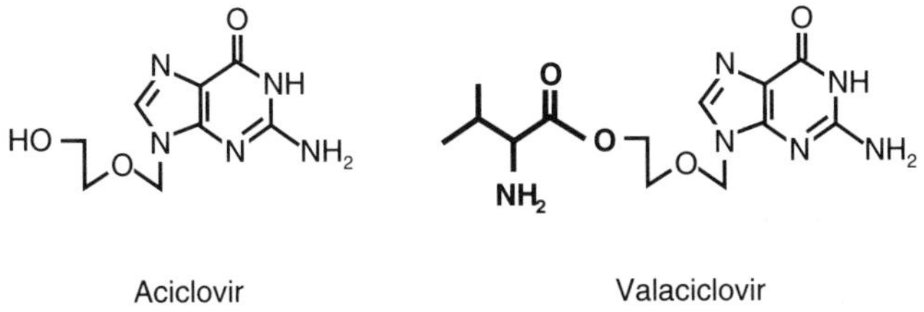

Aciclovir   Valaciclovir

Figure 2.4: Molecular structure of aciclovir and valaciclovir. The amino acid ester of valaciclovir which increases the oral absorption of the molecule is shown in bold.

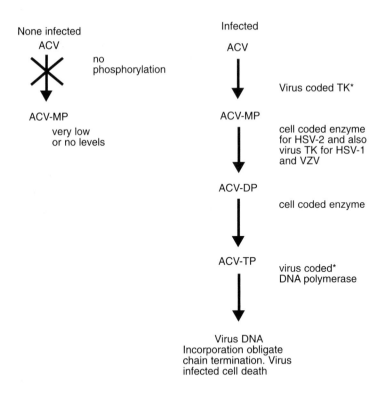

Figure 2.5: Activation pathway of aciclovir in herpesvirus-infected cells.

It is crucial to understand how this mechanism of action allows aciclovir to be a highly potent but selective anti-herpesvirus agent.

- The antiviral activity of aciclovir is caused by the high levels of triphosphate in herpesvirus-infected cells as a result of activating enzymes [in most herpesviruses this is done by the viral coded thymidine kinase (TK) but in the case of HCMV or HHV-6 it is the UL97 gene product. Cellular enzymes do not recognize aciclovir efficiently and hence very low or usually undetectable amounts of aciclovir triphosphate are found in normal cells. This is of importance as the presence of the phosphates of nucleoside analogs may in themselves be toxic to a normal cell.

- The removal of aciclovir from the infected cell pool by synthesis of the triphosphate causes more aciclovir to be drawn into the infected cell. Hence the total concentration of aciclovir and its phosphates in an infected cell is far higher than in a normal cell.

- Finally the viral DNA polymerase utilizes aciclovir triphosphate far more effectively than that of the normal cell leading to inhibition of viral DNA synthesis.

So it is a combination of selective activation plus obligate chain termination that leads to the high potency and safety of aciclovir. It is probably the lack of aciclovir phosphates in normal cells that is the most important factor in safety.

2.9.2 Resistance to aciclovir

Aciclovir is not an antibiotic and the mechanism by which viruses become resistant (albeit rarely) is very different to that of the antibacterials and it is important for the clinician to appreciate this difference. For example, in bacteria resistance is normally coded for by genes carried on extrachromosomal DNA molecules known as plasmids. Genes on plasmids can mutate at a high rate, can associate in groups leading to multiple resistance and can be transmitted from bacteria to bacteria thus spreading the problem. None of these issues are true for herpesviruses and aciclovir. Indeed a recent study on both normals and the immunocompromised can be summarized as follows:

- There has been no net increase in resistant isolates since the introduction of aciclovir.
- The frequency of resistance to aciclovir in the normal individual is very low (0.5%).
- The frequency of resistance in the immunocompromised whilst still being infrequent is higher (ca. 1%) than in 'normals'.

Since the introduction of aciclovir for the treatment of herpesvirus infections the nature of resistant viruses has been studied very closely. Three types of resistant viruses have been identified both in laboratory studies and in the clinic. However, it is also clear that a significant number of isolates obtained from the clinic which are 'not responding to aciclovir therapy' are in fact treatment failures due to inappropriate under-dosing of the compound.

(1) TK deficient— These viruses form the vast majority of clinical isolates genuinely resistant to aciclovir. Such viruses lack all or part of the TK gene that results in low levels of activity. This type of mutant would be expected to be resistant to aciclovir and all other nucleoside analogs. Animal studies show that such TK-deficient viruses are less pathogenic than TK positive viruses. There are very few recorded incidents of clinical transmission of an aciclovir TK-deficient virus. Hence in a normal individual this would be expected to be the basis of negative selection against aciclovir resistance.

(2) TK altered— Viruses which have a mutational change resulting in their inability to phosphorylate aciclovir whilst retaining normal activity with other natural nucleosides. These viruses are the minority of resistant isolates (~10%). They retain the ability to replicate efficiently and also retain their pathogenicity.

(3) DNA polymerase mutations— These involve a mutation in the virus-coded DNA polymerase resulting in its inability to utilize aciclovir triphosphate as a

substrate. Whilst these viruses retain their ability to cause infections they are extremely rare. For example in the 50 million people treated with aciclovir only three isolates resistant to aciclovir due to a mutation in their DNA polymerase have ever been reported.

In the case of HCMV which uses the UL97 gene product to phosphorylate nucleosides, viruses resistant to ganciclovir due to altered UL97 or mutated DNA polymerase have been described. Presumably similar mechanisms exist in the UL97 and polymerase of HCMV to generate viruses resistant to aciclovir.

In conclusion resistance to aciclovir, and presumably other nucleoside analogs, is not of any significant clinical importance in the normal host. In the immunocompromised as the majority of resistant viruses are TK deficient, so the alternative to aciclovir would appear to be a non-nucleoside (albeit with their associated toxicities described below).

Since the discovery of aciclovir clinical trials have shown it to be an effective inhibitor of several herpesvirus infections including those caused by HSV-1 and 2, VZV and to be effective in inhibiting HCMV when given prophylactically. It has an unrivalled safety profile with greater than 50 million patients having received the drug, some for as long as daily for 10 years. In addition whilst not specifically licensed for the management of herpesvirus infections during pregnancy, over 600 pregnant women have been treated with aciclovir with no increased risk of fetal anomalies reported.

2.10 Other antiherpetic agents

There are two connected weaknesses of aciclovir; firstly the relatively low oral availability of the drug in humans (approximately 20%) and a weak activity against HCMV, particularly in treatment of established disease.

For these reasons most efforts to develop alternative therapies for herpesvirus infections have concentrated on treatment of HCMV disease and for drugs with improved oral availability.

2.10.1 Oral availability

There are two alternative drugs now in the process of being licensed for treatment of a variety of herpesvirus diseases. The first is a simple prodrug ester of aciclovir which is called valaciclovir (Valtrex™— also known as Zelitrex™). This compound is an ester of the amino acid L-valine with the aciclovir molecule (*Figure 2.4*). This results in a compound able to deliver by the oral route plasma exposures of aciclovir equivalent to those obtained with intravenous aciclovir. With this derivation, safety has not been a concern and clinical trials have gone on to show that valaciclovir is more effective than aciclovir in the treatment of genital herpes (requiring lower dosing) and zoster infections. Trials are in progress to evaluate its effectiveness in prophylaxsis of HCMV disease.

The second molecule is known as famciclovir (*Figure 2.6*). This molecule is an acyclic nucleoside analog similar, but not identical, to ganciclovir in

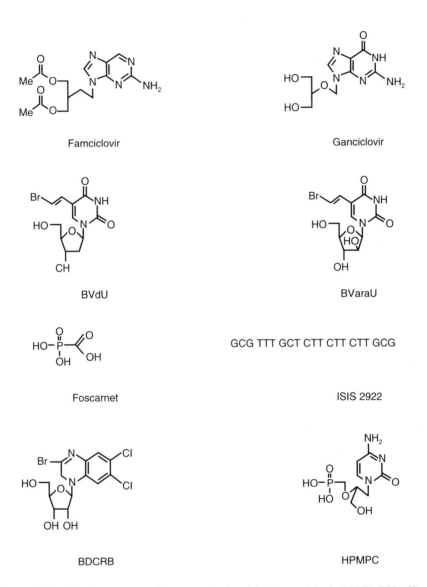

Figure 2.6: Molecular structure of compounds: famciclovir; ganciclovir; BVdU; BVaraU; foscarnet; ISIS 2992; BDCRB; and HPMPC. For full chemical names of these compounds refer to text.

structure. Modification of the moieties shown in *Figure 2.6* occurs after oral uptake and leads to the generation of the parent nucleoside analog penciclovir. Penciclovir has a similar mode of action to that of aciclovir. However, there are some important distinctions from aciclovir that may have an influence on its use in the clinic. The triphosphate of penciclovir has a longer half-life (some 20×) than aciclovir triphosphate. While this in itself may lead to an expectation of better activity for penciclovir than aciclovir it has not been shown in the clinic. The explanation may lie in the fact that, compared to aciclovir, penciclovir triphosphate is a relatively weak inhibitor of the herpesvirus DNA polymerase (160×). Hence these two parameters might be expected to cancel each other out.

One other distinct feature is that penciclovir is phosphorylated to relatively large amounts, compared to aciclovir, in a normal nonherpesvirus-infected cell. This may explain the paradoxical activity of famciclovir against hepatitis B virus. This virus does not code for a thymidine kinase and hence should not be susceptible to any nucleoside analog that is activated with high selectivity by a herpesvirus TK.

Finally the molecular structure of penciclovir and experimental evidence shows that it is not an obligate chain terminator allowing the possibility of incorporation into the growing DNA chain. Indeed in biochemical experiments this has been shown to occur. Chain termination is thought to occur only after the incorporation of multiple penciclovir moieties. Famciclovir is licensed for use in genital herpes and zoster, where it shows similar activity to that of aciclovir.

A third molecule in development is BVaraU (*Figure 2.6*), sorivudine, which was developed as a follow up to BVdU. The arabinoside sugar moiety was developed to stabilize the molecule. Indeed BVaraU has very potent *in vitro* activity against VZV. Unfortunately this activity was not maintained in clinical trials with activity similar to that of aciclovir being found. In addition the drug has a serious contra-indication. In Japan, when given in combination with the anti-cancer nucleoside 5FU, BVaraU resulted in a number of deaths. This was as a result of the inhibition of uracil reductase, by the base of BVaraU, leading to the generation of toxic levels of 5FU. It remains to be seen if this drug will be further developed in Europe and the USA.

2.10.2 HCMV

A number of compounds are in use or in development for HCMV including:

Ganciclovir {[9-(1,3-dihydroxy-2-propoxy)methyl]guanine} (Figure 2.6). This acyclic nucleoside analog, similar in structure to famciclovir is used for treatment and prophylaxis of HCMV disease. Ganciclovir has a similar antiviral profile to aciclovir but is more toxic. One difference between ganciclovir and aciclovir (and penciclovir) is that it has good activity against HCMV. As described above in HCMV-infected cells ganciclovir is phosphorylated by the UL97 product. While this protein has sequences that define it as a protein kinase, both biochemical and genetic studies have shown that it is able to phosphorylate ganciclovir. While detailed biochemical analysis of the ability of UL97 to phosphorylate nucleosides has not yet been reported it is clear that aciclovir is a relatively poor substrate and this may be part of the explanation of the relatively weak anti-HCMV activity of this compound. Mechanistically ganciclovir works in a similar way to penciclovir. That is ganciclovir unlike aciclovir has a pseudo hydroxyl in the 3′ position. While it is clear that DNA replicated in the presence of ganciclovir triphosphate does indeed terminate the mechanism by which it does this is unclear. It may correlate with the cellular toxicity of ganciclovir.

In clinical trials ganciclovir can be shown to be an effective therapeutic for established HCMV disease with responses in the region of 80% depending upon which aspect of HCMV disease is being measured. Upon removal of ganciclovir there is an 80% relapse, and even when therapy is maintained up to 50% of patients relapse, presumably resistance is one factor in this relapse. Ganciclovir has also been shown to have an effect when given prophylactically although there are some studies which do not support this observation.

While showing good anti-HCMV activity its use is limited by its oral bioavailability (now being addressed by the development of an orally active prodrug), bone marrow and spermatic toxicity. These toxicities are limiting, particularly in use in the HIV population, who are commonly treated with a number of other compounds with toxicological problems. In addition, as expected from its mode of action, clinical isolates resistant to ganciclovir with mutations in either their DNA polymerase or UL97 genes (or both) have been identified.

Foscarnet [trisodium phosphoformate (PFA)]–Foscavir (Figure 2.6). This is a pyrophosphate analog and as such is a direct inhibitor of herpesvirus DNA polymerase and does not incorporate into viral DNA as part of its mode of action. Preclinically it has been shown to inhibit a number of viruses including influenza and hepatitis B virus. It does not require phosphorylation by the herpesvirus TK. As it is poorly available by mouth it is delivered by intravenous infusion, it also has a relatively poor penetration across the blood–brain barrier. While PFA is rapidly eliminated from the blood via the urine about 10–30% accumulates in the bone. It has associated nephrotoxicity due presumably to a relatively low selectivity for the viral DNA polymerase. It is important to maintain good fluid levels in patients treated with PFA however, it is of use in HCMV retinitis in AIDS patients. Also since it has an entirely distinct mode of action it has been used in the treatment of herpesvirus infections in those rare cases in which resistance to nucleoside analogs has arisen. However, resistance to PFA occurs in the DNA polymerase of the herpesviruses.

Valaciclovir—Valtrex®. A number of amino acid esters of aciclovir where synthesized in order to increase its oral availability. The optimum compound was found to be the L-valine ester (*Figure 2.4*). Since its metabolism leads to generation of aciclovir and the amino acid L-valine (an essential component of a normal human diet) it was considered to be a safe approach to providing a prodrug. This assumption has been proven correct in clinical trials. The increased oral availability has led to improved activity against HCMV and should lead to a safe effective prophylactic treatment for HCMV disease. Additional benefits have been seen for Valtrex® in treatment of zoster (about 30% improvement in symptoms, especially pain, compared to aciclovir) and genital herpes suppression with a significant improvement in dosing with twice daily administration approved for acute disease treatment and once daily being effective for suppression of recurrent episodes. The clinical studies done so far validate the hypothesis that by increasing the exposure of a patient to aciclovir via administration of valaciclovir a better therapy would be obtained.

HPMPC - Cidofovir (Figure 2.6).   A nucleoside phosphate (*S*)-1-(3-hydroxy-2-phosphonylmethoxypropyl) cytosine-HPMPC is active against a number of herpesviruses, including HCMV, and also nonherpesviruses such as papilloma virus. Since HPMPC it is itself a monophosphate of an acyclic nucleoside analog it does not require herpesvirus thymidine kinase for its activation. It is highly potent against HCMV with selective activity against the viral DNA polymerase of some 1000-fold. Unfortunately this compound shows renal toxicity and while this may be controled by using very infrequent dosing, maintaining hydration and use of probenecid, it will restrict its use. However, it is now licensed in some countries for use against HCMV infection.

1263-BDCRB (Figure 2.6).   This is a benzimidazole with good potency and selectivity for HCMV and a good toxicity profile. It is not clear as to its mode of action but preliminary data suggest that it may be acting against the HCMV UL97 protein. Phase I/II trials are in progress for therapy of HCMV disease.

Anti-sense (Figure 2.6).   An anti-sense oligo nucleoside (ISIS 2922) is in development for HCMV ocular disease. This reagent is based upon a short nucleic acid sequence which may hybridize to an HCMV gene (*IE2*) essential for full virus replication. The hybridization will prevent further transcription of the gene and hence block replication. In cell culture ISIS 2922 is about 30-fold more active than ganciclovir and is active against virus resistant to either foscarnet or ganciclovir. Early indications suggest that it may have promise when used for treatment of HCMV ocular disease where it is administrated by direct injection into the eye. It remains to be determined whether this agent or similar ones will be active when delivered systemically.

2.10.3 Newer approaches

A number of herpesvirus enzymes are currently under investigation as potential targets for antiviral therapy. These include ribonucleoside reductase, thymidine kinase and the herpesvirus protease.

Ribonucleotide reductase.   A conserved gene function in the herpesviruses, this enzyme catalyzes the synthesis of deoxyribonucleosides from their ribonucleosides. The enzyme is comprised of two subunits (so-called large and small) and the requirement for protein interaction has formed the basis of inhibitor design. Peptide, peptidomimetic and small-molecule inhibitors of RR have been synthesized. While these approaches have shown efficacy *in vitro* and in animal models, there is only limited evidence that these agents have any effect on virus in humans. Recently a peptidomimetic inhibitor of RR has been shown to have some effect in topical applications of HSV lesions, but the low oral availability may limit its effect when given orally.

Thymidine kinase.   While the TK of HSV has been shown to be nonessential for replication *in vitro* there is evidence that it is necessary for efficient reactivation of latent virus from neurones. A small number of compounds have been developed as direct TK inhibitors. As yet the poor oral availability of these compounds has limited their effect in animal models, however more recent developments have included the synthesis of orally available prodrugs of TK inhibitors that may have *in vivo* effect.

Protease.   This is a conserved gene function in the herpesviruses which is essential for the synthesis of mature virus particles. Temperature-sensitive mutants of HSV illustrate that the protease is an essential gene function. Many groups have reported the development of high level expression systems for several herpesvirus proteases and assays suitable for screening operations. In addition the enzyme is well characterized biochemically and a high resolution crystal structure has been reported by several laboratories. As yet, however, the work on this target is remarkable by the lack of reports of suitable inhibitors, even early stage.

It is possible over the next few years that compounds with alternative virus targets will emerge. How the alternative 'nonnucleoside' mode of action will translate into clinical properties will be of great interest.

Vaccines.   Over the last 20 years a number of vaccines have been proposed for prophylaxis or therapy of established herpesvirus disease. The history is somewhat confusing with many attempts to use line attenuated, killed or subunit vaccines. Several of these gave good protection in rodent models. However, it is now clear that the rodent models for HSV are not demanding ones and that primates are more representative. Furthermore, the efficacy of subunits was based upon the use of adjutants many of which are not licensed for human use. Currently there is one attenuated vaccine licensed (USA and elsewhere) for use for the prevention of VZV. A number of subunit vaccines are in development for HSV, EBV and VZV disease based upon the use of recombinant protein. Commonly, but perhaps incorrectly, viral glycoproteins have been used as the immunogens. It is notable that one such subunit vaccine for HSV has recently stopped development due to lack of efficacy in clinical trial. A vaccine based upon the EBV glycoprotein gp350 is in early development. If successful this vaccine could have impact on diseases such as IM and also EBV-associated tumors such as Burkitt's lymphoma. In the future it is likely that DNA vaccines for herpesvirus disease will be developed although which virus genes are chosen for such approaches will be crucial.

One possibly more robust approach is the use of a genetically crippled strain of HSV as a therapeutic and perhaps prophylactic vaccine. This approach has the advantage of displaying to the immune system all of the virus proteins in the context of an infected cell, still the most effective method of stimulating cytotoxic T-cell response. One such vaccine using a virus with a deletion in glycoprotein H, essential for fusion of the HSV particle with the target cell, is currently in Phase I clinical trial (*Figure 2.7*). Similar approaches include viruses with deletions in the $\gamma_1 34.5$ gene responsible for CNS replication.

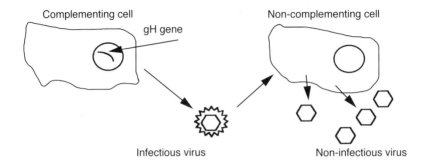

Figure 2.7: Disabled infectious single cycle (DISC) virus. A mutant of HSV is generated by deletion of the gene coding for its glycoprotein H (gH) protein. Glycoprotein H is a structural virus protein which causes virus particles to fuse with cell membranes allowing entry into the cell. In its abscence, the virus particle may attach to the host cell but not fuse and penetrate and hence is not infectious. Production of virus is acheived by the use of a complementing cell line engineered to express gH. Using this cell line, fully infectious HSV may be generated. When this virus is introduced into cells not expressing gH (in the laboratory or in humans), it is able to initiate a full round of replication with all virus proteins (except gH) and produce virus particles which are capable of being released from the infected cell. However, the released particles lack the gH and are in themselves incapable of infecting subsequent cells, limiting the infection. This single round of virus proteins has been shown in animal models to be capable of eliciting a protective immune response and should be ideal as a human vaccine.

It has also been shown that immunization with attenuated strains of HCMV (Towne) may partially protect against HCMV infection in seronegative females with children who attend a nursery. The protection was not considered adequate for a robust vaccine. It is possible that further work may improve this approach to give increased protection. Such a vaccine would have great utility in preventing the possibility of primary HCMV infection during pregnancy, and thus reducing the incidence of congenital disease.

2.11 Conclusion

In the next 5 years the treatment of herpesvirus infections is likely to enter a new phase. The field will build upon the experience with aciclovir. The use of compounds with improved oral availability such as valaciclovir and famciclovir will allow more convenient dosing for diseases such as genital herpes, improved therapeutic effect in diseases such as herpes, zoster and the establishment of effective prophylactic therapy of diseases such as HCMV. A number of specific anti-HCMV drugs will emerge but at present it is too early to say if their selectivity will improve therapy over the existing potent but toxic compound ganciclovir. Some additional compounds with alternative modes of action may emerge. Several vaccines both therapeutic, and perhaps prophylactic, will be produced which may have significant effect on herpesvirus disease. Finally it is likely that a number of rapid diagnostic systems (perhaps family doctor based) will be produced in the next few years. These should allow a more dependable diagnosis of herpesvirus disease and the use of therapeutics with more effect. For the clinician the prospect of such developments can only be encouraging.

Further reading

Fields, B.N., Knipe, D.M. and Howley, P.M. (eds) (1996) *Fields Virology,* 3rd Edn. Lippincott-Raven, New York, pp. 1787–2062.

Johnson, S. and Johnson, F.N. (eds) (1996) Anti herpes virus agents. *Reviews in Contemporary Pharmacology,* **7** (2), 13–19.

Chapter 3

Chemotherapy of human immunodeficiency virus infections

3.1 Introduction: AIDS and human immunodeficiency virus

3.1.1 AIDS

Barely 15 years have passed since the first hints of a new disease arose in North America in the early 1980s. The initial manifestations were the appearance in otherwise healthy young men of illnesses previously restricted to entirely separate epidemiological groups. For example, Kaposis' sarcoma, (KS) had been found almost exclusively in elderly males from the southern Mediterranean until the incidence of cases in California and New York began to accelerate in 1981/82. Since then we have come to recognize and classify the symptoms and the clinical aspects of acquired immunodeficiency syndrome (AIDS) in great detail, as described in a previous volume in this series [1].

3.1.2 The aetiological agent

The pattern of opportunistic infections associated with this new disease, such as pneumocystis carinii pneumonia (PCP), CMV retinitis, or mycobacterial infection, hinted at a generalized immunodeficiency. Flow cytometry established that the acquired immunodeficiency was consistent with pronounced depletion of CD4$^+$ helper T cells from the normal level of about 1000 per mm^3 of blood to fewer than 200. In addition, the pattern of transmission within risk groups, hinted at a sexually transmitted infectious agent. The viral agent causing AIDS was quickly identified by Montagnier and Gallo, in 1983, as a new human retrovirus. Initially this virus was called adult T-cell leukaemia virus (ATLV/Montagnier) or human T-lymphotropic virus type III (HTLV III/ Gallo) but is now known as human immunodeficiency virus (HIV).

Furthermore, HIV showed marked tropism for CD4$^+$ T cells and macrophages and gave rise to early suggestions that the loss of CD4$^+$ cells in AIDS patients was the result of direct cell lysis *in vivo*. Given that only some 2–3% of CD4$^+$ T cells appear to be infected with HIV even at late stages of full-blown AIDS, then additional mechanisms of CD4$^+$ T cell depletion were proposed. This included destruction by HIV specific CD8$^+$ cytotoxic T cells, T cell anergy/ apoptosis-priming by 'soluble' viral envelope proteins, or HIV induced CD4$^+$ T cell redistribution from blood to lymph nodes. However, recent data from Shaw and Ho [2,3] have shown that levels of CD4$^+$ T cells rise rapidly after reduction in levels of plasma HIV by drug therapy, suggesting that the loss of CD4$^+$ T cells is directly linked to HIV replication.

3.1.3 Cytokines and disease

In addition to the loss of cellular components of the immune system, soluble factors have emerged as key regulators of AIDS progression. Several HIV sero-positive individuals failed to develop full-blown AIDS within the expected 10–12 year timeframe, and close studies of these individuals suggested release of a soluble protective factor. This soluble factor appeared to be released from the CD8$^+$ T cells of these long-term nonprogressors, and one component was thought to be new cytokine IL-16, a lymphocyte chemoattractant factor (LCF). Anecdotal evidence suggested that IL-16 prevented HIV infection of CD4$^+$ T cells by binding directly to and blocking the CD4 receptor molecule on the surface of these cells. As the CD4 receptor was also the receptor for initial HIV binding (see below), then IL-16 directly excluded HIV binding to CD4$^+$ T cells. However, when the 'CD8 factor' was identified it contained a cocktail of β-chemokines (chemotactic cytokines), including MIP1α, MIP1β and RANTES, but not IL-16. Almost simultaneously with the identification of the soluble factors, the elusive second receptor for T-cell adapted HIV was identified as the LESTR chemokine receptor, dubbed 'fusin' and now known as CXCR4. A different chemokine receptor, CCKR5, was identified as the second receptor for primary HIV strains that display tropism for macrophages. The inhibitory effects of these chemokines almost certainly result from their physical blocking of HIV binding to its co-receptor. Elevated levels of β-chemokines are thought to contribute to the natural resistance of 'at risk' individuals to HIV infection. Moreover, human genetic studies have established that members of the same cohort of long-term nonprogressor have mutations in the gene for CCKR5 that render the receptor defective; as these individuals developed normally, it raises the real possibility that CCKR5 is a viable anti-HIV target molecule [4,5]

Stimulation of CD4$^+$ T-helper cells by antigen results in the production of distinct patterns of lympokines. The T helper 1 response (T_h1) is generally associated with cell-mediated immunity and viral clearance involving the lymphokines interferon γ (IFN-γ) and IL-2, whereas the T helper 2 response (T_h2) is associated with humoral immunity and tissue/organ inflammation in response to IL-4, IL-5 and IL-10. Healthy HIV-seropositive individuals appear to mount a T_h1 response to

HIV infection characterized by large numbers of antiviral cytotoxic T lymphocytes (CTL/CD8+) whereas during progression to AIDS, the helper T-cell subset (CD4+/CD7+) associated with T_h1 cytokine production declines while the T_h2 T-cell subset (CD4+/CD7-) increases. This T helper switch may contribute to the disease patterns seen with late stage opportunisitc infections where very poor cell-mediated responses are mounted to 'endogenous' pathogens, such as HCMV and pheumocystis.

The role of HIV-suppressing and HIV-inducing cytokines has been well reviewed recently [6].

3.1.4 Dynamics of virus replication and disease

The pattern of clinical latency, where a person can be HIV positive for a long time (10–12 years) before showing any symptoms of AIDS, appeared to correlate with an extended period of proviral latency during the HIV replication cycle (see below). However, re-consideration of earlier data together with a new finding based on quantative polymerase chain reaction (PCR) assays show that HIV is never truly latent. The level of HIV in the blood plasma has been shown to vary over several logs from the acute stage of infection to the onset of full-blown AIDS. What is now clear is that the virus is replicating at all times and at a remarkable rate. Studies from David Ho and George Shaw demonstrated that as much as 30% of plasma virus is replenished daily; for a typical HIV-1 infected individual, this amounts to 100 million virions per day (this number has since been revised upwards to an average of 10 000 million virions per day). These studies also gave some hope for antiviral therapy (see below), and rekindled the as yet unresolved debate as to whether direct CD4+ cell killing by HIV was entirely responsible for the eventual decline in this cell population [2,3,7].

Recent data have shown that the various lymph nodes of the secondary lymphoid system, rather than circulating peripheral blood mononuclear cells (PBMCs), are the major reservoirs of HIV. Ho and Shaw observed that when virus replication was suppressed by antiviral drugs, the levels of blood CD4+ T cells rose rapidly at a rate of about 5% of total CD4+ cells per day. One viable explanation for this rapid rise in cell numbers is the redistribution of CD4+ cells from the lymph nodes. Taken together with data showing that levels of HIV in lymph nodes are very high, then the source of the plasma HIV is probably T cells from the lymph nodes. Virus-expressing cells in the lymph nodes would initially be trapped by follicular dendritic cells (FDC), but it has been thought for some time that continuous HIV replication brings about gradual immunologically mediated destruction of FDCs. Gradual loss of lymph node architecture, through loss of FDCs, facilitates greater release of HIV-infected T cells and accounts at least in part for the rise in plasma HIV as AIDS develops [7].

The high rates of virus replenishment also provide the perfect milieu for generation of HIV mutants. With pressure from anti-retroviral therapy, these mutants evolve drug resistance.With pressure from the immune system, CTL escape mutants evolve. These latter mutants develop insensitivity to cytotoxic

T cells through alterations in *gag* or *gp120* peptide sequences that are normally immunodominant targets for MHC class I presentation. A third type of mutant virus has been recognized for several years, one in which the V3 loop of *gp120* is altered so that the virus goes from a nonsyncytium inducing form (NSI) to a syncytium inducing form (SI). Syncytia are giant multinucleated cells that form when viral proteins on the outer membrane of infected cells lead to fusion with membranes of uninfected cells. SI forms are better able to spread locally, particularly in the presence of neutralizing humoral immunity, through cell-to-cell transmission and are known to replicate at considerably enhanced rates in T cell cultures. These considerations have lead to the proposal that the strategy for anti-HIV chemotherapy should be to hit HIV, early and hard [8].

3.1.5 Vaccines

Virus replication in cells of the immune system and at high levels renders the development of HIV vaccines daunting, particularly when it is clear that a good CTL response to the acute phase of HIV infection offers no protection during later stages of disease. There are numerous vaccine candidates, including subunit vaccines, peptides and DNA, being developed (at least 14 currently) but, with the exception of Remune from the Salk Institute, none have made it into Phase III clinical trials. A growing appreciation of HIV immunopathology, together with new funding initiatives from the US National Institutes of Health and the Rockerfeller AIDS Vaccine Initiative, has also lead to resurrgent interest in developing vaccines, particularly those that will induce a mucosal immunity at the main portals of viral entry, together with humoral and cell-mediated immunities [9].

3.1.6 Clades/geographic distribution

The *ad hoc* group determining the taxonomy of HIV recognized that two types of HIV had been found: HIV-1 which is associated with North American and European AIDS, and HIV-2, identified by Clavel and Montagnier, in 1986, which is associated primarily with AIDS in West Africa. More recently, HIV-1 has been sub-classified into 10 alphabetical subtypes, or clades, including one orphan clade (Clade 0), that relate to the phylogenetic clustering of viral envelope or gag nucleotide sequences (*Figure 3.1*). To date most work has been performed on HIV-1 from the B clade, for example LA1, but as levels of AIDS increase in developing countries and other subtypes appear in Western nations, an awareness for the need for therapeutics to be effective against HIV-1, and all its clades, plus HIV-2 is increasing.

3.2 HIV replication

3.2.1 Retroviruses

Although we have known about HIV and its role in AIDS for only 15 years, retrovirus-associated disease has been recognized for the best part of the 20th century,

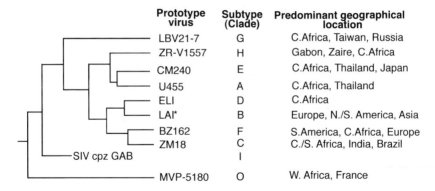

Prototype virus	Subtype (Clade)	Predominant geographical location
LBV21-7	G	C.Africa, Taiwan, Russia
ZR-V1557	H	Gabon, Zaire, C.Africa
CM240	E	C.Africa, Thailand, Japan
U455	A	C.Africa, Thailand
ELI	D	C.Africa
LAI*	B	Europe, N./S. America, Asia
BZ162	F	S.America, C.Africa, Europe
ZM18	C	C./S. Africa, India, Brazil
SIV cpz GAB	I	
MVP-5180	O	W. Africa, France

Figure 3.1: The HIV-1 subtypes (clades) are shown together with the geographical location in which they predominate. Prototype members of each subtype are shown and their phylogenetic linkage indicated. Chimpanzee SIV (Gabon isolate) is shown for reference. LAI* is one of the clade 'B' viruses that are used in drug screening assays.

for example Rous sarcoma virus (RSaV) and malignant disease in chickens, equine infectious anemia virus and equine swamp fever. The first human retrovirus identified was human foamy virus (HFV) in 1971, but the first retrovirus associated with human disease, human T cell leukemia virus type 1 (HTLV-1), was discovered in 1980. Myoshi and co-workers were first to link HTLV-1 with the adult T cell leukemias that were prevalent in geographic pockets of Japan. Within three years, Montagnier and Gallo demonstrated a retrovirus was associated with AIDS; this was given the agreed name of human immunodeficiency virus (HIV) in 1986.

The retrovirus family is divided into simple and complex viruses based on the number of proteins expressed from the provirus. Both simple and complex retroviruses express at least three major gene products called gag (Group specific Antigen), pol and env (*Figure 3.2*). The gag and env polypeptides are components of the virus particle. Processing of the gag precursor produces the capsid proteins, which in the case of HIV includes p24 ^{gag}; the appearance of p24^{gag} in serum is the very first signs of HIV infection. Processing of env gives rise to the transmembrane (TM) and surface (SU) glycoproteins; for HIV the precursor env protein is gp 160 and the products are known as gp41 (TM) and gp 120 (SU) (*Figure 3.2*). The pol gene product is processed to produce the 'replicative' enzymes: protease, reverse transcriptase, RNasH and integrase. This group of enzymes were the first, and are still the best, targets for anti-HIV chemotherapy. As a complex retrovirus, HIV also encodes at least six so-called 'auxiliary' or accessory gene products which, although small polypeptides (9–27 kD), have often-complex regulatory functions (*Figure 3.2* [10]). Three of these polypeptides, tat (increases provirus transcription), rev (increases cytoplasmic level of unspliced env mRNA) and nef (alters CD4 levels on the surface of infected cells and alters virus pathogenicity) have been exploited as targets for anti-HIV therapy and are discussed below. The

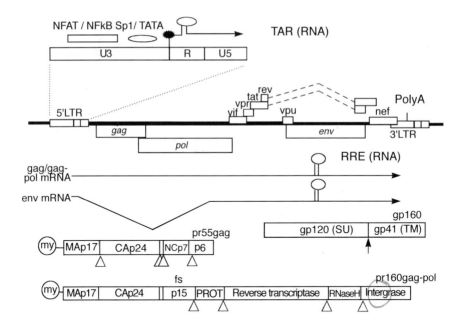

Figure 3.2: The HIV-1 genome with open reading frames (ORFs) is shown. The major retroviral genes, *gag, pol* and *env* are shown in boxes below the genome and auxiliary gene products are shown above the genome. Tat and rev are spliced regulatory products as indicated by dashed lines linking the two ORFs (see text for details). PolyA indicates region on 3′ LTR that serves as signal for polyadenylation of genomic and messenger mRNA. The left most LTR (5′ LTR) is shown expanded to indicate the regions in U3 that are bound by regulatory transcription factors such as nuclear factor of activated T-cells (NFAT) and nuclear factor kB (NFkB) and by core transcription factors such as Sp1 and the TATA box binding proteins. Transcription initiation at the boundary of U3/R is shown by star, mRNA containing the TAR element is shown by arrow with bubble. The major mRNA species encoding gag, gag–pol and env are shown below genome, with splicing of env mRNA plus location of the RRE element indicated. The protein products of these mRNAs are shown at bottom, with precursor polypeptides above box and mature products within the box l(see *Table 3.1* for details). GP160 is cleaved by host cell serine protease at one site (↑) whereas pr55^{gag} and pr160$^{gag-pol}$ are cleaved by the viral aspartyl protease at eight sites (△).

remaining three accessory proteins, Vpr, Vif and Vpu, may become feasible therapeutic targets as more information is gathered on their functions [10]. Currently, Vpu (9 kD) is thought to enhance release of virus particles from infected cells, partly through its ability to bind to and release CD4 and CD4–gp160 complexes in the endoplasmic reticulum, allowing gp160 processing to gp120 and gp41 and degrading CD4. Vpr (15 kD) enhances virus yield from infected cells by first facilitating transfer of the HIV pre-integration complex to cell nuclei, a property shared with MA protein, and secondly by locking infected cells in the S–G$_2$ phase of the cell cycle, resulting in greater virus yield and suppression of CTL-mediated apoptosis. Finally, Vif, a 23 kD virion structural protein, enhances the ability of HIV to initiate infection, possibly by aiding transport of virus particles to cell nuclei via vimentin rich intermediate filaments. It may also have a role in the information of proviral DNA as a result of 'stabilizing' replicative intermediates following first and/or second strand synthesis. The degree of inhibition of HIV replication that may be gained through inhibition of Vpr, Vif or Vpu has not been established, and so they will not be discussed further. The HIV gene order and expression pattern are depicted in *Figure 3.2*, and the functions of HIV proteins are summarized in *Table 3.1*.

3.2.2 Binding, entry and uncoating

The HIV env proteins gp120 and gp41 are linked noncovalently on the surface of HIV particles, with gp41 responsible for the fusion of cell and viral membrane following binding of particles to target cells. 'Identification' of target cells for infection by HIV is mediated by the interaction of gp120 with its specific receptor, the CD4 molecule that is found predominantly, but not exclusively, on the surface of T-helper cells. Since T-helper cells are depleted in AIDS patients, then a very obvious association between HIV infection and immunodeficiency was formed in 1984 by David Klatzman, Robin Weiss and co-workers. However, therapies based on soluble CD4 molecules or CD4–toxin conjugates failed because clinical, that is, nonlaboratory adapted, strains display variable affinities for CD4. This variable affinity probably exemplifies the range of minor variants that compose the HIV 'quasispecies' which evolve during development of AIDS in each individual.

The presence of a second receptor was recognized when it was shown that not all cells expressing CD4 could be infected by HIV, and it is this second receptor that may offer a better target for antiviral therapy. The gross change in tropism from macropage/monocytyte preference to T-helper cells appears to be associated with the switch from the NSI to SI phenotype. This results from changes in the gp120 variable loops 1,2 and 3 (V1, V2, V3) which alter the selectivity for the chemokine receptors, from CCKR5 to CR4. There is evidence that binding of gp120 to CD4 induces a conformational change in gp120 that increases its interaction with CCKR5. As discussed above, mutations in CCKR5 are associated with natural resistance to macrophage-tropic HIV, but have no apparent effects on the individual. Therefore, antiviral therapies utilizing small molecules that block CCKR5, in a manner akin to the inhibitory chemokiness MIPα, MIPβ and RANTES, could provide safe and effective HIV therapies aimed at the pre-eminent (macrophage-tropic) variant. A number of assays are running against the chemokine receptors and leads from these screens may well show efficacy (*Figure 3.3*, inset).

Occupancy of the chemokine receptors alters membrane polarity thus assisting gp41-mediated fusion of the viral membrane with the cell envelope. Peptidic and nonpeptidic fusion inhibitors have been identified, but peptides have pharmacological problems whereas the early nonpeptidic inhibitors were associated with considerable toxicity *in vitro* and *in vivo*. Therefore, only one fusion inhibitor,

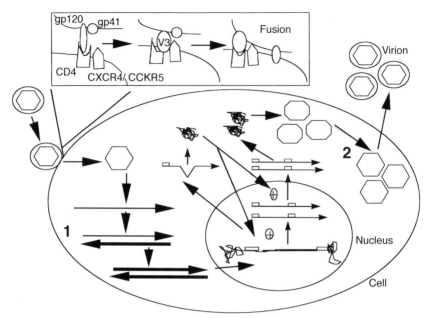

Figure 3.3: The viral life-cycle is depicted, with the binding and fusion events involving gp120 and gp41 fom the virus and the two receptors on the cell surface of macrophages (CD4/ CCKR5) or T-lymphocytes (CD4/CXCR4) shown in expanded view. The replication cycle proceeds from left to right, with reverse transcription (1) leading to integrated provirus in nucleus of cell. The provirus first expresses spliced regulatory products, containing TAR element only. These regulatory products then facilitate ($\oplus$) nucleocytoplasmic translocation and translation of structural gene products (gag, pol and env) with protease (2) mediating maturation of capsids. Acquisition of an envelope from the cell membrane during budding gives extracellular infectious virion. Processes (1) and (2) are the targets of currently licensed drugs for inhibition of reverse transcriptase and protease, respectively.

pentafuside, has progressed into clinical trials. As such inhibitors would be particularly useful against SI variants of HIV in patients with advanced disease, the results of these trials are eagerly awaited.

3.2.3 Reverse transcription and integration

The early stages of the replication cycle, binding and uncoating, and the late stages, viral protein synthesis, assembly and budding, are all typical of a generalized virus replication cycle (*Figure 3.3*). However, retroviruses produce an enzyme, called reverse transcriptase (RT), that is largely unique, with the exception of hepatitis B virus (Chapter 5) and the mobile genetic elements called retrotransposons. Hence, RT makes an ideal target for antivirals. RT is carried within the incoming virus capsids, which are released into the cytoplasm of the infected cell following cell–virion fusion. HIV RT is a heterodimeric RNA-dependent DNA polymerase consisting of a p66 and a p51 subunit. The enzyme is initially synthesized as a p66 homodimer, but processing by the HIV protease enzyme (*Figure 3.2*) releases a 15 kD protein from one subunit, and the remnant p51 subunit undergoes a marked conformational change. This conformational change was appreciated following determination of the structure of HIV RT to 2Å resolution in 1995 — the same primary amino acid sequence gives rise to markedly different secondary protein structures. RT catalyzes copying of the single-stranded RNA genome into double-stranded DNA via a RNA–DNA hybrid. The RNA component of this hybrid is removed by ribonuclease H (RNaseH) activity associated with the RT; the RNaseH structure has also been solved (in 1991) but no inhibitors of this activity have yet been identified. Formation of the double-stranded DNA from the genomic RNA all takes place within the cell cytoplasm in an 'open' form of the viral capsid called the pre-integration complex. This pre-integration complex is extremely stable ($t_{1/2}$ of 16 h) but like all complex retroviruses, and unlike simple retroviruses, contains short peptide sequences, called nuclear localization signals, which facilitate nucleo-cytoplasmic transfer of the complex in the absence of mitosis (*Figure 3.3*).

Once inside the cell nucleus, another unique retrovirus encoded enzyme, called integrase (IN), catalyzes the insertion of the double-stranded DNA intermediate, known as the provirus, into the genome of the host cell. This 288 amino acid enzyme is cleaved from the C-terminus of RT in the gag–pol polyprotein by the HIV protease (see below) and is carried into infected cells within the viral capsid. Its activities include both the 3′ processing of the dsDNA intermediate, whereby two nucleotides are removed adjacent to a conserved CA dinucleotide, and DNA strand transfer, where following cleavage of the target phosphodiester bond, the CA-OH3′ is inserted into the host cell genome. These activities can be mimicked using recombinant enzymes and screening systems for inhibitor identification have been set up (see section 3.5.1).

3.2.4 Provirus expression

This integrated DNA copy of retroviruses, called the provirus, is transcribed into messenger RNA (mRNA) by cellular RNA polymerase II, giving initially a number of spliced mRNA species, but following *de novo* synthesis of rev, unspliced viral mRNAs also appear in the cytoplasm for translation. As with all retroviruses, the integrated provirus is stable and when the cell divides, it segregates with the host cell chromosomes and can thus be transmitted from cell to cell without viral replication. This form of the virus cannot be attacked by antiviral agents until it becomes transcriptionally active in response to, for example, cytokines such as IL-2 and TNFα which activate the NKkB transcription factor. Transcription of the provirus and translation of the mRNA utilizes cellular enzymes, although, as noted above, the complex retroviruses augment these cellular enzymes with their own transactivators. At the junction of the provirus with the host cell DNA are DNA elements known as long terminal repeats (LTR; see *Figure 3.2*) arranged in the pattern U3-R-U5. The LTRs are derived from the 5′ end (R-U5) and the 3′ end

(U3-R) of genomic viral RNA during reverse transcription, and because of their location relative to the coding regions of the provirus, serve different functions in the regulation of virus expression. The 5′ LTR binds specific and general transcription factors that regulate the initiation of mRNA synthesis, whereas the 3′ LTR signals the point at which mRNA synthesis should end with addition of the polyA tail. In respect of these different functions, the 5′ LTR has been the subject of considerable analyses, and regulatory elements and binding sites for more than a dozen transcription factors have been identified. The real surprise, however, was the discovery that HIV-1 and HIV-2, and subsequently most of the complex retroviruses, encoded additional transcription factors that enhanced mRNA production from the 5′ LTR.

The first HIV-1 encoded transcription factor recognized is called tat (for **T**rans**A**ctivator of **T**ranscription). A variety of experiments identified precisely the gene for tat and also the target sequence for tat, called TAR (**T**rans**A**ctivation-**R**esponse element). Deletion of the *tat* gene from proviral clones reduced the infectivity of the clones to undetectable levels, and recent data has shown that *tat⁻* viruses are transmitted in cell culture about three orders of magnitude less well than *tat⁺* viruses. These data, showing that tat was essential for virus growth and transmission, suggested that tat and its interaction with TAR were targets for anti-retroviral drugs. The full length HIV-1 tat polypeptide is 86 amino acid long and is encoded by a spliced mRNA of two introns and three exons (*Figure 3.2*). The first exon is noncoding, the second exon encodes amino acids 1–72, and the third exon amino acids 73–86. Two forms of tat have been found in infected cells; tat 1–72 was as active as tat 1–86, but there is some evidence that tat 1–86 is better able to activate HIV LTR sequences integrated into host cell chromosome and also env mRNA which contains a second, TAR-like element.

The tat protein contains a basic amino acid motif RKKRRRQRRR, which by its nature was expected to bind nucleic acid, and on the basis of shared homology with phage anti-terminator proteins, the ligand was expected to be RNA. This was confirmed when TAR was shown to be a bulged RNA stem-loop. Tat binds specifically to TAR RNA *in vitro* with the basic domain, and in particular arginines R-52 and R-53, contributing from the protein and uridine-23 in the bulge contributing from the RNA ligand to this specificity. The structure of the tat basic region and of TAR RNA have been solved separately by 3D-NMR, and although the interaction of tat and TAR RNA has been studied by circular dichroism, high resolution images of the tat–TAR RNA complex are awaited. Intercalators have been identified which interact with TAR RNA with high affinity, and some inhibit tat binding, but one as yet have shown an appreciable therapeutic index separating anti-HIV activity from cytotoxicity. Owing to its location within the U5 region of the HIV LTR, TAR is present in all HIV RNA species.

Tat also has some extracellular activities which include growth factor-like stimulation of Kaposis' sarcoma (KS) cells, angiogenesis of KS lesions, neurotoxicity, and cell exit and cell uptake of transactivation-competent tat protein. The reproducibility and relevance of these activities to AIDS pathogenesis are unresolved at present and so will not be discussed further.

3.2.5 Processing, maturation and release

HIV and many other retroviruses, including RSaV, use virus-encoded protease enzymes to chop up the two long precursor proteins, gag and gag–pro/pol, into the mature proteins. These mature proteins then come together to form a shell around viral RNA molecules, that are also transcribed from the integrated provirus, and eventually this shell (or capsid) passes into and through the host cell membrane. During this final process, the virus capsid acquires part of the host cell membrane that includes a third major viral protein, env. The presence of env in the membrane of the virus is the key to selective infection of cells in the next round of virus replication because env recognizes receptor proteins on the surface of specific cells (*Figure 3.3*).

Table 3.1 summarizes where known, the function of individual HIV-1 proteins.

Table 3.1: Function of HIV gene products

Gene	Precursor	Products	Functions/Comments
gag	p55 gag	p17 MA*	Matrix protein connecting lipid envelope to capsid
		p24 CA*	Major structural protein that multimerizes to form virus capsid
		p7 NC*	RNA binding nucleocapsid protein that condenses RNA into virion
		p6	Poorly defined function but appears to affect virus release along with VPR
gag–pol	p160 gag–pol	p17 MA*	As above
		p24 CA*	As above
		p15	Fusion protein formed by frame-shifting; function unknown
		PRO**	10 kD aspartyl protease that cleaves gag & gag-pol precursors
		RT**	Encodes 66 kD and 51 kD components of reverse transcriptase heterodimer
		RNaseH**	Inactive 15 kD fragment cleaved from one p66 polypeptide to give p51
		INT**	20 kD integrase enzyme; catalyzes insertion of DNA provirus into host cell genome
env	gp160	gp120 SU*	Extracellular component of viral envelope; forms trimeric structure, binds CD4, chemokine 2nd receptor
		gp41 TM*	Membrane spanning component of envelope; responsible for virus fusion
tat		TAT***	15 kD transcriptional activator, interacts with TAR RNA element & host transcription factors; extra cellular activities, e.g. as Kaposis growth factor
rev		REV***	Mediates cytoplasmic appearance of viral mRNA containing RRE RNA element
nef		NEF***	Involved in signaling via src homology (SH3) region; down regulates CD4; increases virion infectivity
vif		VIF***	Increases infectivity of virus in peripheral blood cells & some T-cell lines
vpr		VPR***	Arrests cells in G2 phase of cells cycle
vpu		VPU***	HIV-1 specific; down regulates CD4 expression
vpx		VPX***	Specific to HIV-2; function not known

* Structural proteins.
** Replicative enzymes.
*** Regulatory/ auxiliary functions.

3.3 RT inhibitors

3.3.1 AZT (zidovudine)

The unique enzymatic activity of reverse transcriptase (RT) is an obvious target for anti-retroviral therapy, and indeed current HIV therapy hinges on a RT inhibitor, azidothymidine (AZT). AZT was originally synthesized as an anticancer drug in 1964, and was also investigated in experiments with avian and murine retroviruses. Further studies showed that HIV was inhibited by AZT and this efficacy was observed in small clinical trials in 1985/86, leading to the rapid development of AZT for anti-HIV therapy. AZT inhibits virus growth because, after phosphorylation by cellular enzymes to AZT-triphosphate (AZT-TP), RT recognizes AZT-TP in place of the normal nucleotide triphosphate, deoxythymidine TP (dTTP), and incorporates it into the growing strand of DNA. However, AZT cannot form the normal 3´-to-5´ phosphodiester bond with the 5´ hydroxyl group (5´-OH) of the next nucleotide to be incorporated because the key 3´-OH group on the ribose sugar has been replaced by the azide group (see Chapter 1). Thus elongation of the growing DNA chain is terminated. Two other lisenced therapies for HIV are also chain terminators that target RT, and both, dideoxyinosine (ddI) and dideoxycytidine (ddC), have the 3´ hydroxyl group replaced by a hydrogen atom (*Figure 3.4*).

The best developed inhibitors of HIV, AZT, ddC and ddI, were discovered by moderate throughput live virus screening assays, and RT was subsequently shown to be the target by a variety of molecular studies. None the less, the novel activity of this enzyme and its key role in HIV replication ensures that RT remains a key target for antiviral therapy. In the clinic AZT was shown to be effective for the treatment of advanced HIV disease, although side-effects of the drug (primarily anemia and neutropenia) were quite severe in some individuals.

3.3.2 Other nucleosides

In addition to the dideoxynucleoside inhibitors, ddI (didanosine) and ddC (zalcitabine), two other nucleosides, d4T (stavudine) and 3TC (Epivir) have been proven to have durable activity against HIV RT to the extent that they are lisenced therapies (*Figure 3.4*). Both d4T and 3TC are chain terminators by virtue of a 2´–3´ double bond or 3´ sulfur, respectively, and show good antiviral activity *in vivo*. Another carbocyclic nucleoside similar to carbovir, known as 1592U, showed weak activity *in vitro*, but was shown to be a potent inhibitor of HIV *in vivo*. 1592U has also been shown to effectively cross the blood–brain barrier, making this drug particularly valuable in the treatment of AIDS dementias [1,4,6]. All three show resistance mutations that are distinct from AZT (see below) and indeed the mutations associated with high level (1000-fold) 3TC resistance, M184^V/$_I$, confer suppression of resistance to AZT. Phosphorylation of the nucleosides to the phosphorylated forms is undertaken entirely by cellular enzymes because HIV, unlike some of the herpesviruses, does not encode a nucleoside kinase. Attempts to overcome the potential lack of selectivity because of the absence of a viral kinase include production of monophosphate prodrugs such as POM-PMEA

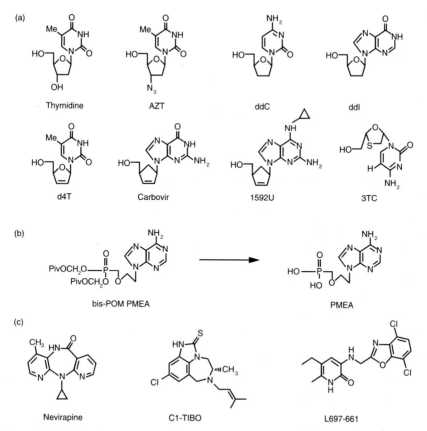

Figure 3.4: (a) The first three licensed therapies for HIV are shown in the first line together with thymidine, and its natural ribose sugar, for reference. Newer nucleoside RT inhibitors are shown in the next line. Note that the sugar residue in 3TC is in the L-configuration rather than the natural D-configuration. (b) Shows the production of active inhibitor (PMEA) from its more soluble prodrug (bis-POM PMEA). (c) Examples of the most advanced and widely used nonnucleoside RT inhibitors. See text for details.

(*Figure 3.4*), a more bioavailable and quantitatively metabolized form of phosphonyl methoxy eythyl adenine (PMEA). All nucleosides are now considered largely for combination therapies and so pharmacological parameters, such as the site or severity of toxicity or penetration of the CNS, may determine utility as much as antiviral activity.

3.3.3 Nonnucleoside RT inhibitors (NNRTIs)

Live virus screening assays and structure–activity relationships (SARs) lead to the discovery of a second type of RT inhibitor, the nonnucleoside RT inhibitors (NNRTI), exemplified by nevirapine, C1-TIBO and L-697,661 (*Figure 3.4*). The triphosphates of the nucleoside inhibitors were shown to be competitive inhibitors of recombinant RT activity and appeared, therefore, to bind into the catalytic site of the enzyme. However, all the NNRTIs were shown to be noncompetitive inhibitors of the recombinant enzyme, and so their binding was assigned to an 'allosteric' site with influence on the catalytic site. These latter enzymological observations were of importance when crystallographers were searching for ways to enhance RT crystal formation. Almost all NNRTIs to date give rise rapidly, that is in days rather than weeks, to high level resistance, >1000-fold, both *in vitro* and in patients. The rate and level of the emergent resistance is due to one key alteration, the mutation Y181C[1]. However, in combinations with nucleoside inhibitors, resistance to NNRTIs has not emerged, due certainly to the drug cocktails suppressing HIV replication to extremely low levels, and so the NNRTIs certainly have clinical utility (see below).

3.3.4 Inhibitor design

It proved to be a relatively straightforward task to express the HIV reverse transcriptase p66 in *E. coli* with the added benefit that the enzyme was cleaved in *E. coli* extracts during purification to an equimolar mixture of p66 and p51 subunits. This p66/p51 heterodimer is the form of RT observed in virions, where processing of the p66 homodimer to hetrodimer in infected cells is carried out by HIV protease. This cleavage releases an RNaseH domain (15 kD), assumed to be inactive. *In vitro* studies established that the p66/p51 heterodimer was significantly more active than the p66 homodimer.

In 1992, two groups solved the structure at moderate resolution (3–3.5 Å). The group led by Steitz solved the RT structure to 3.5 Å resolution by incorporating the NNRTI, nevirapine, whereas the structure derived by Arnold *et al.*, at 3.0 Å resolution used an anti-RT monoclonal antibody sub-fragment and a DNA oligonucleotide to enhance enzyme rigidity. The structures confirmed the suspected asymmetry of the hetrodemeric enzyme, in that p66 and p51 adopt very different conformations despite having an identical amino acid sequence, and the path of the RNA/DNA template through the central cleft, or palm, of the enzyme between the 'fingers' and 'thumb'/RNaseH domains. Although the Steitz structure was able to show that nevirapine interacted with residues Y181 and Y188, thereby preventing enzyme flexibility and rationalizing the Y181C mutation that renders HIV>100-fold resistant to nevirapine, the limited resolution made it difficult to produce fully refined structures adequate for inhibitor design. However RT crystals produced by David Stammers and David Stuart diffract to approximately 2 Å [11]. Again, the enzyme structure was stablized by incorporation of a NNRTI similar to nevirapine. These high resolution structures offer an opportunity to design RT inhibitors of similar potency to those designed to inhibit HIV protease, and given the clinical success of RT inhibitors, there is a real hope that an effective therapy for AIDS might arise from this work.

---

[1] The one letter code for amino acids is used throughout. Generally, the letter relates to the first letter of the corresponding amino acid. There are these exceptions to the code: R = arginine, N = asparigine, D = aspartate, Q = glutamate, E = glutamate, K = lysine, F = phenylalanine, W = tryptophan and Y = tyrosine.

3.3.5 Resistance

Clinical trials in patients with advanced HIV disease showed that AZT provided clinical benefit for periods of 6–12 months, but subsequently the benefits declined, and CD4 cell levels, a surrogate measure of HIV disease progression, fell to pre-therapy levels with a concomitant increase in viral p24 levels. Brendan Larder [12] showed that virus from patients who had received extensive AZT treatment had decreased sensitivity to AZT, and subsequently went on to show that specific mutations were associated with this altered sensitivity. These mutations, M41L, K67N, K70R, T215Y and K219Q, were able to confer various degrees of AZT resistance, depending on individual or multiple combinations, when introduced by site-directed mutagenesis into an isogenic infectious proviral clone. Levels of resistance ranged from 4-fold with one mutation (M41L) to 180-fold with four mutations (M41L/K67N/K70R/T215Y). Unlike the situation with recombinant HIVprotease, where virus resistance mutations results in resistance at the enzyme level (see below), recombinant RT did not show resistance in a variety of assay conditions. Therefore, with AZT resistance it has been difficult to demonstrate that changes the sensitivity of RT to inhibition is the cause of viral resistance, and the hope is that crystallographic studies might offer insights into this discrepancy (see below).

Presently, at least 14 drugs, or drug groups, active against RT have given rise to resistance mutations under selection pressure in cell culture. The general notion is that nucleoside inhibitors tend to give lower levels of resistance, than NNRTIs, and that while high level resistance with NNRTIs, >100 fold, may involve only one mutation, high level resistance to nucleotide inhibitors requires two or more muta-tions. There are exceptions, of course, and 3TC, a nucleoside, gives >1000-fold resistance with one mutation (M184$^V/_I$), whereas L-697,661, a non-nucleoside inhibitor, shows only 2–8-fold resistance with individual mutations. In addition, resistance development tends to be very rapid with NNRTIs as their site of action lies outside the active site and may be mutationally less constrained. One very interesting development from the resistance work with these various inhibitors is the observation that certain mutations that confer resistance to one drug, for example MI84V for 3TC or L74V for dd1, may suppress the phenotypic effects of other mutations, such as those responsible for resistance to AZT. These observations suggest that there may be novel ways of combining RT inhibitors to slow the development of resistance (see below). Recently, solution of the structure of mutant enzyme, co-crystallized with the selecting inhibitors, has provided atomic detail of RT drug resistance. *Table 3.2* summarizes most of the known RT resistance mutations.

Viruses incorporating amino acid changes in RT, arising from inhibitor selection, tend to grow less well than parental virus when the drug selection is removed. However, some mutant viruses, for example K70R, do grow almost as well as parental viruses.

Table 3.2: Resistance mutations for RTI, NNRTI and PRI

Selecting drug	Key mutation(s)	Fold resistance	In vivo	Cross resistance	Auxiliary mutations	Comments
(A) RT inhibitors						
AZT	M41L	4	Y		T215Y	41 + 215 mutations give 60× resistance
	D67N		Y		M41L,K70R,T215Y	Quad mutant 180× resistance
	K70R		Y		K67N,T215Y,K219Q	Quad mutant 120× resistance
	T215Y/F		Y			T215Y reversed by L74V (ddl), Y181C (NNRTI), M184I/V (3TC)
	K219Q					As part of quad gives 120× rsistance
ddl	K65R	4 - 10	Y	ddC		
	L74V	5 - 10	Y	ddC		Reverses AZT resistance
	M184V	2-5×	Y	ddC, 3TC		Reverses AZT resistance mutations
ddC	K65R	4 - 10	Y	ddl		
	T69D	5×	Y	ddl, 3TC		
	L74V	5 - 10	Y	ddl, ddC,		
	M184V	2 - 5	Y	ddl, ddC		
d4T	V75T	7	Y	ddl, ddC	M184V	8× resistance
1592U	K65R	3	Y	ddl, ddC	M184V	9× resistance
	L74V	4	Y	ddl, ddC, 3TC	L74V,Y115F	11× resistance
	M184V/I	3	Y	ddl, ddC		Mutations suppress AZT resistance
3TC	M184V/I	>100	Y	3TC, ddl, ddC		Suppresses AZT resistance
PMEA	K65R	7 - 25	?	3TC		
	K70E	9	?			Confers 2× susceptibility to PFA
(B) NNRTI						
Nevirapine	V106A	100	Y	Other NNRTIs		Can suppress AZT mutations
	Y181C	>100	Y	L697-661		
cl-TIBO	K103N	>100	Y	L697-661		
	Y181C	>100	Y	Cl-TIBO		
L697-661	K103N	8	Y	Other NNRTIs		Many other muations found but 103 and 181 most common
	Y181C	>30				
(C) Protease inhibitors						
Ro31-8959	G48V	2	Y		A71V, I84V	Rare *in vivo*
	L90M	5	Y			Frequent *in vivo*
L735-524	V32I		Y	A-77003	M46L, V82A	Triple 3× resistance
	M46I/L		Y		V32I, A71V, V82A	Quad is 14× resistant
	L63P		Y		L10R, M46i, V82T, I84V	Quin is 8× resistant
	V82A/F/T		Y			Combination to get 8 - 14× resistance
ABT-538	V82A	2 - 6	Y	XM323, ABT538	K20R,M36I,I54V	Quad is 41× resistant
	V82T	2 - 6	Y	XM323, L735-524	K20R,M36I, I54V,A71V	Quad is 28× resistant
VX-478 (141W94)	I50V	2	?		M46,I47V	Triple is 10-20× resistant
AG1343	D30N	7	Y		D88N	Double is 8× resistant
	A71V	5	?		D30N	Double is 7× resistant
	I84V		?	many PRI	M46I,L63P,A71V	Quad is 30× resistant
XM323	V82A/I/F	2		some PRI	M46I,L97V	Triple is 11× resistant
	I84V	12		many PRI	V82F	Double is 92× resistant

3.4 Protease inhibitors

3.4.1 From enzyme assays

Expression of the protease region of HIV in *E.coli* produced active enzyme which cleaved radiolabeled HIV gag precursor at specific sites. HIV protease recognizes at least eight cleavage sites in the gag and gag/pol precursor, the latter formed by transitional frame-shifting and the location of these specific sites and their amino acid sequences are shown in *Figure 3.2.* Inhibition of the HIV protease in *E.coli* allowed production of sufficient enzyme for purification, enzymatic characterization and crystallization. Enzyme overexpression also contributed to protease inhibitor design by the more traditional route of structure–activity relationships (SARs). Once expressed and shown to be active, small oligopeptides comprising 4–8 amino acids were used to define the optimum substrates for the enzyme. This information was then used in two ways. Firstly, in inhibitor design, where particularly potent substrates were modified so that the 'scissile' bond, that is the peptide bond where the enzyme cleaves the peptide, was so modified so that it was no longer cleaved. Substitutions, known as isosteres, such as hydroxyethylene and hydroxyethylamine, gave rise to the licensed inhibitors L-735,524 (indinavir) and Ro31-8959 (saquinavir) (*Figure 3.5*). Secondly, cumbersome HPLC-based assays for peptide cleavage, were replaced by more rapid peptide based assays that incorporated chromogenic, fluorogenic or radiolabeled groups into the side chains of optimized peptides. The readout from these groups was altered by cleavage, and so inhibition of cleavage could also be simply detected. Using such assays, mass screening with recombinant protease was undertaken, which allowed discovery of novel inhibitors, for example penicillins variants, or active members of compounds selected for complimentarity to the HIV protease active site, for example haloperidol. The symmetry of the protease structure and a symmetrical dihydroxy-ethylene isostere gave rise to the C_2-diols, and the best members in this series were identified by rapid screening. However, even this information may not be enough to generate potent systemic antivitals. Abbotts' A-77003 proved to be a very potent antiviral agent in the test-tube, but failed in the clinical trials due largely to poor pharmacokinetics. More bioavailable follow-up compounds to A-77003, identified by protease, viral and pharmacokinetic screening, such as ABT-538 (ritonavir; *Figure 3.5*), are now licensed.

3.4.2 From enzyme structure

The crystal structure showed that HIV protease was an almost symmetrical dimer. Soon after the solution of the apo-enzyme structure the structure of chemically synthesized protease was solved, both as an apo-enzyme and as a 'holo' enzyme binding one of the first inhibitors of HIV protease, called MVT-101. This showed that a region of the protease dimer, called the flap and comprising residues 43–58, closed over the top of the inhibitor, locking into place within the enzyme active site. Movement of the flap was the most dramatic rearrangement observed but

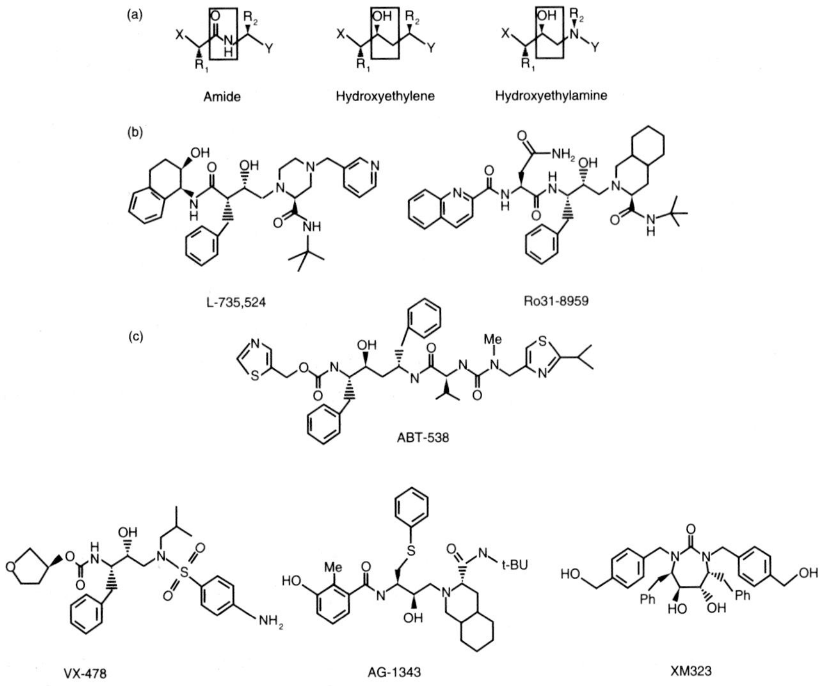

Figure 3.5: (a) Depiction of the natural site for proteolysis (amide bond) together with isosteres based on the intermediate form of the cleavage site. (b) Licensed inhibitors of HIV protease based on these isosteres. (c) Inhibitors in late stages of development that were derived from structure modeling. XM323 is no longer in development but is also a prototype of the structure-based inhibitors.

other minor changes showed that the symmetry of the apo-enzyme was lost. This indicates a way for the symmetrical enzyme to accommodate substrates that were not symmetrical. Since the first structure determinations in 1989, more than 200 structures of proteases with inhibitors bound have been solved and can be studied at various sites on the World Wide Web.

Of course, the purpose of these structural determinations was to aid the design of potent inhibitors of HIV to help combat AIDS, and one of the best examples of the exploitation of this information are the cyclic urea derivatives designed and synthesized by DuPont Merck. The prototype of this class, XM323 (*Figure 3.5*) had subnanomolar activity against the enzyme and submicromolar activity against the virus. The purpose of the central unit, the actual cyclic area, is beautifully simple. The two hydroxyl groups (-OH) interact with the two catalytic apartate residues, D25 and D125′, and the single carbonyl substitutes for the 'flap water', found in the MVT-101:protease structure, forming hydrogen bonds with residues I50 and I150′ to lock the enzyme shut and inactive. The branch chains out of the central unit were then designed to fill the side pockets of the protease dimer, normally occupied by amino acid residues of the protein substrate, to provide enhanced binding affinity. XM323 has inhibitory activities against protease and HIV that are 10- to 100-times better than inhibitors developed from SARs. So structural information holds great promise for anti-HIV therapy, but the trade-off is that the spectrum of anti-retroviral activity may be diminished, that is AZT inhibits many retroviruses but has only moderate anti-HIV activity, whereas XM323 is very potent against HIV but has very weak, or no, activity against other retroviruses. Molecular modeling has given two HIV protease inhibitors, Nelfinavir (AG-1343) from Agouron and VX-478 from Vertex/ Glaxo Wellcome, that are currently in the latter stages of clinical development (*Figure 3.5*).

3.4.3 Resistance to protease inhibitors

The emergence of viruses resistant to RT inhibitors during chemotherapy and the progression of protease inhibitors into clinical trials, prompted many groups to search for resistance to protease inhibitors. For all inhibitors tested in cell culture, resistant variants of HIV have arisen under drug selection. Once the link between virus resistance and protease sensitivity is established — and such a correlation is not always possible in the case of resistance to RT inhibitors — then overexpression of the key mutant enzymes and crystallography allows the atomic definition of resistance.

In most examples of resistance to inhibitors, the structure of the inhibitor bound into the wild-type enzyme is known. Computer modeling packages then allow substitution mutagenesis 'on-screen', and the results are often sufficient to explain resistance. For instance, modeling of the V32I mutation, which appears in response to the inhibitor A-75925, suggests a decrease in the size of the pocket normally occupied by the valine residue of the inhibitor, thus decreasing the binding affinity. A similar model was proposed for the mutation V82I responsible for resistance to A-77003. However, when John Erickson and A. Wlodawer determined the structure of V82I enzyme with A-77003 bound, they found that their model was only half right [13]. Only one monomer actually bound the side chain of the inhibitor as poorly as predicted, while the second monomer accommodated the mutation by altering its structure, that is, the mutant enzyme possessed more asymmetry than wild-type enzyme. One comforting observation is that most viruses carrying protease resistance mutations, as is the the case with the majority of mutations in RT, grow substantially less well than parental HIV in cell culture. However one mutant with the L90M change, associated with resistance to saquinavir, and some mutants selected with ritonavir do grow at least as well as the parental strain. The incapacity of the mutant virus is a direct result of diminished protease activity.

3.5 Other targets for chemotherapy

3.5.1 Integrase

The activities of the intergrase enzyme can be assayed *in vitro* using oligonu-cleotide mimics of the unintegrated proviral termini, and enzyme expressed in *E.coli* is active in such assays. This then opened the doors for selective screening of topoisomerase inhibitors, DNA binding agents, and other nucleic acid inter-calating agents, several proving to have anti-integrase activity. For example, the anti-tumor agent, NMHE, had an IC_{50} (concentration for 50% inhibition) of 1 μm, doxorubicin an IC_{50} = 1–2 μm, and aurintricarboxylate (ATA) monomers an IC_{50} = 10 μm. The ATA monomers also showed moderate anti-HIV activity of 30 μm. Oligonucleotide-based inhibitors of integrase, such as Aronex's AR-177, have been given to a small number of patients, but have not been developed further to date. Combinations of such active compounds with inhibitors of other targets (RT, protease) may be useful in suppression of HIV replication. AZT-monophosphate (AZthymidylate) also inhibited integrase at high concentrations (IC_{50} = 150 μ), suggesting that AZT antiviral activity may include a contribution from integrase inhibition. The structure of the catalytic core of the integrase (aa50–212) was solved in 1995, and so this enzyme could also become a target for modelers and drug designers. Finally, a macrophage/monocyte-derived protein has been identi-fied which binds specifically to the integrase; this interaction could also be a tar-get for inhibition if it proves to be essential for virus replication. Preventing inte-gration could be a significant advance as it reduces the frequency of stable chemotherapeutically 'invisible' proviruses; it is this feature of HIV replication that may make a cure extremely difficult.

3.5.2 RNase H

Recombinant RNaseH activity can be obtained from expression in *E. coli* by inclusion of 60 or so residues N-terminal of the cleavage site separating p51 and RNaseH. Unfortunately, to our knowledge, no inhibitors of HIV replication have been obtained from RNaseH enzyme assay-based screening or from inhibitor modelling based on the structure.

3.5.3 Tat

For some time, there was no *in vitro* functional assay for tat activity, and so screen-ing assays looked at the transactivation of a LTR-linked marker enzyme by tat expressed from a plasmid, or recombinant tat protein added to cell culture medi-um, or looked directly at the tat binding to TAR RNA *in vitro*. The Roche group were the first to identify small molecule inhibitors of tat function through trans-fection screening. These inhibitors, Ro5-3335 and Ro24-7429, belong to the chemical class of benzodiazepines, which also includes diazepam and other anti-depressants, an area in which Roche has excelled for many years. These inhibitors were effective against HIV in both acute and chronic infections in cell culture, and both progressed as far as preclinical and clinical phase I trials. However, in these trials, they showed no anti-viral activity, as monitored by p24 and CD4 cell levels, and both showed a degree of toxicity. Attempts to define the activity of Ro5 and Ro24 showed that they did not prevent the tat–TAR interaction, but could stop tat transactivation of using *in vitro* transcription assays. In addition, they stopped tat transactivation when added to cell culture medium, and stopped tat effects on translation in frog oocytes, all of which suggested that there was no effect on tat synthesis but rather an effect on the interaction of a cellular polypetide with tat and/or TAR RNA. This conclusion was supported by the failure to generate viruses resistant to the inhibitors by passage in cell culture, and by the development of *in vitro* transcription assays that showed enhanced tat activity in the presence of the RNA polymerase II transcription factors TFIIF and TFIIS.

These *in vitro* functional assays also showed that cellular TAR RNA binding proteins also enhanced tat activity, and since several of these cellular proteins also function in the regulation of host cell translation, the narrow therapeutic window of Ro5 and Ro24 may be due to the inhibition of cellular translation as well as tat-activated virus transcription. Keto/enol epoxy steroids also inhibit tat transactivation of LTR-marker plasmids, and HIV replication, but again the therapeutic window proved to very narrow.

Currently, the most promising tat inhibitors are a series of short basic peptides developed by Allelix, with the lead compound of this series, Alx40-4c, in phase II/III clinical trials. Studies of short peptides binding to TAR RNA showed that a stretch of nine arginine residues bound to TAR RNA with the higher affinity than a peptide containing the wild-type *tat* basic domain, RKKRRQRRR, and the R9 peptide competed and challenged wt peptide from TAR RNA. As the R9 peptide also worked in *in vitro* transcription assays, transfection assays, tat cell uptake assays and in acute and chronic HIV replication assays, then only poor pharmacokinetics and stability tempered further development. The amino acids were altered from the normal L-stereoisomer to the D-isomer, and this D-peptide, Alx40-4c, showed greater stability but still potent anti-HIV activity. Modified forms of tat-derived basic peptides, called peptoids, where the arginine side chain is moved from the α-carbon to the nitrogen of the amino acid, have also been shown to inhibit tat, and their development as anti-HIV drugs may be feasible.

3.5.4 Rev

Rev, the **R**egulator of **E**n**V**, was the second novel HIV regulatory activity found by transient assays and by RNA blotting and hybridization. It was known that HIV expressed three classes of mRNA, of approximately 2, 4 and 9 kb (including full-length genomic RNA), with the 2 kb mRNA class having at least two large introns, the 4 kb class one large intron and 9 kb class apparently being unspliced. Subsequent experiments have shown that although HIV encodes only nine or ten gene products, there are about 30 different mRNA species that are derived from splicing events using primarily six splice acceptors and two splice donors. In the absence of rev (which was then known as the trs gene product), HIV was not able to express normal levels of the gag and env proteins, and this effect was due to the absence of the 4 and 9 mRNA classes from the cytoplasm of infected cells. Transient assays mapped the *trs* gene to a region overlapping the *tat* gene, and also mapped two elements in the 9 kb RNA species that were involved in post-transcriptional regulation of gag and env expression. These elements were called crs (**cis-re**pression sequences) and car (**cis a**ctivation **r**egion), indicating that one element, car responded to rev whereas the other, crs, acted independently of rev. Crs is now known as INS (instability sequences) and make unspliced cytoplasmic RNA a target for rapid degradation, whereas car was renamed the RRE (rev response element) and was subsequently shown to specifically bind rev. The RRE sequence is approximately 300 bases long, and appears to fold into a complex secondary structure containing several double stranded stems with varying length single strand loops. It is located within the env open reading frame and initial binding of RRE by rev occurs at a very high affinity site in stem-loop II. This binding is a nucleation point for subsequent lower affinity, cooperative binding by more rev monomers which may eventually result in rev coating large regions of the 4 and 9 kb RNA species. This binding is thought to suppress splicing by masking splice donor/accceptor sites, or facilitate nucleo-cytoplasmic transport of unspliced RNA, or prevent recognition of INS (or all three). The net effect is that stable unspliced gag and env RNA species appear in the cytoplasm and get translated.

Since viruses unable to express active rev protein are not infectious, then rev would appear to be valid target for chemotherapy. Two rev-specific processes make good molecular targets for intervention; the initial binding to RRE and multimerization of rev. The multimerization step can be inhibited by mutant rev proteins that have a 'transdominant phenotype', and the best example is a rev variant isolated by Malim and Cullen called M10. Studies with M10 confirmed that inhibition of rev multimerization resulted in the inhibition HIV growth, and even most clinical isolates of HIV are inhibited by M10 protein. Gene therapy trials have begun in the USA where M10 protein is introduced into cells by retroviruses and results are awaited.

Three small molecule inhibitors of rev have been reported and all affect the binding of rev to its high affinity sites. The most promising inhibition was by neomycin B which was able to inhibit HIV replication in chronically infected cells. The therapeutic window was small however, possibly due to poor uptake by cells in culture. The intercalating dye, pyronin Y, inhibited rev binding, but was cytotoxic in cell-based assays, and major groove binding agents, such as bis-piperidines and bis-piperazines, have yet to be tested for antiviral activity. In all cases, there is clearly the need for development of more effective inhibitors based on these initial leads. Our own experience has shown that many agents which bind to RRE and TAR RNA do not display any great selectivity, and as a result are highly cytotoxic in HIV assays. The structure of TAR RNA, and the impending solution of the structure of RRE stem-loop II, may make it possible to design and synthesize selective inhibitors, particularly if the structures include bound ligand.

3.5.5 Nef

Of all HIV proteins, nef is the most enigmatic. Initially identified as a 15 kD protein in the HXBc2 strain, full-length nef from other strains, when expressed in *E. coli,* was shown to be a mixed species of 25 and 27 kD with associated GTP-binding and GTPase activity. However, few groups have been able to reproduce these activities, and so initial biochemical assays have not materialized. In transient transfection assays using mammalian cells, nef was shown to down regulate the HIV LTR through a short sequence known as the NRE (**n**egative **r**esponse **e**lement) and hence the name, nef (for **ne**gative **f**actor) seemed appropriate. Yet few groups have been able to reproduce this effect, so no transient assay for nef function has been developed.

Two separate lines of research lead to some indication of nef function and the effects of this activity. Firstly, animal studies with Simian immunodeficiency virus (SIV), as described below. Secondly, it had been known for many years that HIV infection of CD4 T cells in PBL cultures lead to a reduction in the levels of the CD4 marker expressed at the cell surface, as monitored by FACS analysis. The HXBc2 strain, which has a truncated nef, did not induce this lowering of CD4 levels. This implied that nef was responsible for this down-regulation, but attempts to demonstrate direct interactions between nef and the CD4 marker uniformly failed. However, it was subsequently shown that recombinant nef will bind directly to CD4 but only if nef is myristolated and as such bound to cell membranes. Previous studies with *E. coli* expressed nef probably failed because bacteria are unable to suppport such post-translational modifications of recombinant proteins. The interaction of nef with CD4 has the potential for an assay for nef function. Recently, it has also been shown that nef interacts with proteins containing src homology 3 (SH3) domains. Thus direct monitoring of interactions, or by using surrogate measures of protein–protein interactions such as the yeast two hybrid system, in molecular screening programs may identify inhibitors of nef interactions with CD4 or SH3. As virus variants lacking nef, either through truncation or deletion, still grow well in cell culture, there is no quick way of demonstrating antiviral activity for nef inhibitors.

The true effects of nef inhibition may only be seen in animal models, because studies of SIV in macaques were the first to demonstrate a role for nef in viral pathogenesis. Desrosier, and now Stott, showed that animals infected with SIV variants lacking nef function did not develop disease as rapidly as animals infected with wild-type virus. Animals surviving wild-type virus inoculation showed deletion or alteration of nef whereas animals succumbing to disease after inoculation with nef⁻ viruses showed reversion of nef to wild-type sequence. It has also been shown, however, that nef⁻ viruses cause disease in neonatal macaques at high innoculation doses. Therefore, while the purpose of down-regulation of CD4 would appear to be prevention HIV-superinfection of already infected cells, especially significant given the new insights into the dynamics of HIV replication and T-cell replenishment, quite how this relates directly to the experiences with SIV and monkeys is not fully understood.

3.5.6 CD4/gp120

Modified versions of the CD4 molecule, the receptor for HIV gp160/120 were being developed as inhibitors of virus binding (Stage 1; *Figure 3.1*), virus budding and for targeting of cytopathic toxins. However, the failure of recombinant CD4 to bind to clinical strains of HIV led to the abandonment of this strategy. More recently, synthetic peptides derived from the complementarity determining region 3 (CDR3) of CD4 domain D1, constrained by cyclization, inhibited lab strains of HIV-1. As these peptides also impaired CD4/MHC class II function and almost certainly will not be active against clinical variants of HIV, they will be unlikely to make viable drugs.

3.6 Novel approaches

3.6.1 RNA-based inhibitors

Anti-sense RNA, that is RNA species with complimentarity to specific viral mRNAs resulting in formation of double-stranded RNA which are then digested by cellular double-strand specific ribonucleases, have been developed to target both gag and tat mRNA and are currently in phase I/II trials. Ribozymes, that is RNA molecules capable of catalyzing the site-specific cleavage of specific viral mRNA, have also been developed for gene therapy of HIV infection and are undergoing safety evaluation. In addition, RNA decoys containing multiple copies of the TAR RNA target for tat have been developed. More recently small RNA molecules, or aptamers, selected by the ability to bind to chosen target molecules, irrespective of the function of that target molecule, have been proposed as viable inhibitors of HIV replication, but so far none have been developed with sufficient potency to merit further development.

As infant, and therefore, unproven technologies, these four RNA-based approaches are unlikely to gain widespread acceptance beyond small scale 'proof of principle' studies; a quantum leap in efficacy and/or delivery technologies will be required before small-molecule or other biotechnological approaches are usurped.

3.6.2 Gene therapies

As discussed above, gene therapy trials have begun with the rev M10 transdominant mutant, although no data is available at present. There are many ideas for anti-HIV gene therapies, including approaches that use 'attenuated' HIV vectors as CD4$^+$ T-cell or macrophage-monocyte specific delivery vehicles. For detailed technical discussion of these approaches, reference should be made to Drupolic and Jeang [14].

3.6.3 Immunomodulation

Recombinant immunomodulators have also been proposed as anti-HIV therapies, largely as adjunctive therapies to small-molecule antivirals [15]. For example, recombinant interleukin 2 (IL-2) has been proposed as a therapy to induce replication of all integrated HIV proviruses, particulary of species are that are transcriptionally silent (*sic* latent). Once all proviruses in all body compartments are activated in this way, traditional antivirals are used to eradicate these viruses and the cells producing them. Killing of infected cells would also be mediated by cytotoxic T-cells, which would also be activated by the IL-2 therapy. However, such novel therapies clearly have immense risks that counterbalance the theoretical benefits of 'curing' individuals of latent HIV. Biocon have proposed using an IL-2 agonist as a safer and more effective adjunctive therapy than IL-2 itself.

3.7 Combination therapies

3.7.1 Combinations in the clinic

Recent data from David Ho [7] and others, showing that a triple drug combination could lower plasma viral RNA titers to below detectable levels for prolonged periods of time, has prompted considerable excitment. Part of the excitement relates to the calculation, as a result of this sustained antiviral activity, of the half-lives of 'long lived' viral reservoirs and extrapolation of these half-lives to suggest that HIV could be totally eradicated from infected individuals in about 3 years. There are patients approaching their second aniversary on these triple combinations and so we should begin to access data quite soon indicating whether 'cure' is an appropriate term for HIV disease. Triple combinations that are in progress all include the combination of AZT and 3TC, together with either a protease inhibitor (including VX478, ritonavir and nelfinavir) or a NNRTI (including both nevirapine and MKC-442). Therefore, single pill formulations of optimum doses of AZT and 3TC are being produced and will form the cornerstone of triple and quadruple combinations.

In addition to the antiviral activities of these combinations, some consideration does have to be given to the pharmacological/ toxicological effects of such long-term treatments. The accidental but none the less lethal combination of sorivudine and 5FU during anti-herpes chemotherapy is ample warning. For instance, saquinavir, indinavir and ritonavir all interact with the liver cytochrome P450 isoenzymes, and so combinations of these inhibitors may not be viable for this reason. A number of NNRTIs also interact with the same liver enzymes again perhaps limiting the possibility of using some protease inhibitors with, for example, nevirapine. Conversely, it has been shown that co-administartion of ritonavir elevates levels of saquinavir, and so careful monitoring of liver metabolism and responses therein, may actually derive some benefit to patients.

3.7.2 Sequential therapy vs. concurrent therapy

A number of *in vitro* studies have shown that two anti-HIV drug combinations provide an effect that is greater than the sum of the two individual components, giving a synergistic response. Other combinations can give an inverse synergy or antagonism, and are unlikely to be of value in the clinic. However, synergistic drug interactions *in vitro* may help determine combinations of value should pharmacotoxicology be suitable. Examples of this are AZT and 3TC and AZT and NNTRIs, both of which gave strong synergy that extrapolated to enhanced antiviral activity in patients. Interestingly, protease inhibitors combined with nucleoside RT inhibitors have also given synergy (e.g. VX478 and AZT; saquinavir and ddC) as have two protease inhibitor combinations. Such observations provide evidence in favour of concurrent combination therapies.

However, Brendan Larder and others have shown that there are instances where a resistance mutation for one drug renders a virus, previously resistant to a second drug, sensitive to that second drug again. Examples of this are documented with the reversal of AZT resistance by mutations associated with ddI resistance (I74V) and 3TC resistance (M184I/V), as well as nevirapine and other NNRTIs. Therefore, cycles of monotherapy may be as effective as dual therapy, although current clinical practice clearly favors triple or quadruple combination therapies administered as early as possible following evidence of seroconversion. In addition, the observation that monotherapy always leads to development of resistance and that the mutations arising may confer resistance to other inhibitors in addition to the selecting agent probably precludes sequential drug monotherapies. Cross-resistance is a particular problem with NNRTIs, for example Y181C selected by nevaripine will also be resistant to many other NNRTIs . Cross-resistance has also been observed with protease inhibitors and is a common feature of the mutations arising after monotherapy, for example the M46I/L63P /A71V/I84V virus selected with nelfinavir is also less sensitive to both indinavir and saquinavir.

3.8 Conclusions

The complexity of HIV replication and the nature of the disease that it causes has provided a challenge to academic and industrial scientists alike. The challenge has been to provide medicines that suppress HIV replication but also permit reconstitution of the immune system back to its preexisting homeostasis. With a greater appreciation of the natural history of HIV infection, particularly the sustained and rapid turnover of virus and T cells alike, and an increased understanding of the immunopathological effects, resulting in part from the widespread loss of immune function, successful antiviral therapies are in place and new immunotherapies are in development. However, these therapies, the result of multidrug cocktails and/or complex biotechnological products, remain prohibitively expensive for under developed nations where the real problem of HIV infection now lies. In addition, we must broaden our therapies to non B clades of HIV-1 and also to HIV-2. The challenge into the year 2000 and beyond is to produce affordable, effective therapeutics while developing strategies for prevention of HIV transmission. So, despite some very exciting progress in the last few years in our battle with HIV, there is no quarter for complacency. The problem of global HIV disease still exists. On a brighter note, while many therapies are developed with HIV and AIDS in mind, the spin-offs for gene therapy, biotechnology and chemotherapy of other viruses and diseases are immense and should not be underestimated either.

References

1. Nye, K.E. and Parkin, J.M. (1994) *HIV and AIDS*. Bios Scientific, Oxford.
2. Perelson, A.S., Neumann, A.U., Markowitz, M., Leonard, J.M. and Ho, D.D. (1996) *Science*, **271**, 1582.
3. Wei, X., Ghosh, S.K., Taylor, M.E., Johnson, V.A., Emini, E.A., Deutsch, P., Lifson, J.D., Bonhoeffer, S., Nowak, M.A., Hahn, B.H., Saag, M.S. and Shaw, G.M. (1995) *Nature*, **373**, 117.
4. Fauci, A.S. (1996) *Nature,* **384**, 529.
5. Wain-Hobson, S. (1996) *Nature*, **384**, 117.
6. Antia, R. and Halloran, M.E. (1996) *Trends in Microbiology,* **4**, 282.
7. Perelson, A.S., Essunger, P., Cao, Y., Vesanen, M., Hurley, A., Saksela, K., Markowitz, M. and Ho, D.D. (1997) *Nature*, **387**, 188.
8. Ho, D.D. (1995) *N. Eng. J. Med.*, **333**, 450.
9. Kennedy, R.C. (1997) *Nature Medicine,* **3**, 501.
10. Miller R.H. and Sarver, N. (1997) *Nature Medicine*, **3**, 389.
11 Ren, J., Esnouf, R., Garman, E., Somers, D., Ross, C., Kirby, I., Keeling, J., Darby, G., Jones, Y., Stuart, D. and Stammers, D. (1995). *Nature Structural Biology*, **2, Q4.**
12. Larder, B.A. (1996) in *Antiviral Drug Resistance* (D.D. Richman, ed.). John Wiley & Sons Ltd, Chichester.
13. Wlodawer, A. and Erickson, J.W. (1993) *Ann. Rev. Biochem*, **62**, 543.
14. Dropulic, B. and Jeang, K-T. (1994) *Human Gene Therapy,* **5**, 927.
15. Pantaleo, G. (1997) *Nature Medicine* **3**, 483.

Further reading

Blair, E.D. and Darby, G. (1996) in *The Molecular Biology of HIV/AIDS* (A. Lever, ed.). Wiley, Chichester, p.159.
Challand, R. and Young, R.J. (1996) *Antiviral Chemotherapy*. Spektrum GmbH, Munich.

Chapter 4

Chemotherapy of respiratory virus infections

4.1 Introduction: diversity of viruses associated with respiratory infections

Respiratory viruses, by definition, include all viruses that are transmitted via the respiratory route and replicate in and destroy cells in the surface respiratory epithelium leading to local respiratory disease symptoms. Extensive damage to the protective ciliated columnar epithelium occurs but is frequently localized to certain regions of the respiratory tract, depending on the infecting virus, which give rise to certain disease syndromes. For example, in the common cold (rhinitis) the nasal passages or anterior nares in the upper respiratory tract are affected, while in influenza damage is more extensive with the lower respiratory tract involved, typically the larynx, pharynx, trachea and bronchi. Frequently different viruses produce similar disease symptoms, and the same virus is able to cause variable respiratory syndromes. The main aim of chemotherapy of respiratory infections is to inhibit virus replication and limit the damage to the respiratory epithelium and as a result reduce the acute symptoms but also prevent the longer term symptoms which may arise due to respiratory impairment.

Grouping viruses based on disease syndrome means that morphologically distinct viruses are grouped together. There are five families (viridae) of viruses, indicated in *Table 4.1*, that contain viruses which may be classified as respiratory viruses, namely, orthomyxoviruses, paramyxoviruses, picornaviruses, coronaviruses and adenoviruses. In *Table 4.1* the disease syndromes associated with each virus group are listed with the most common ailments in bold. Other virus families may be associated with respiratory disease, but generally cause other disease syndromes, or respiratory disease may be associated with immunological suppression, for example, many of the herpesviruses.

Viruses with RNA genomes are responsible for the vast majority of acute respiratory disease. Since the RNA viruses are capable of high mutation rates, presumably because their RNA polymerases are error prone and lack error correction facilities, there is considerable phenotypic diversity in the surface antigens within the virus groups associated with respiratory disease. Thus, antibody pressure

Table 4.1: Viruses causing respiratory disease

Virus group	Virus structure	Serotypes	Disease syndrome
Picornaviruses	ssRNA,+ve sense, nonsegmented genome, nonenveloped		
Rhinovirus		1A,1B, 2-101	**rhinitis (common cold)** pharingitis
Coxsackie		A21, A24	pharingitis, rhinitis
Echoviruses		11, 20	rhinitis
Coronaviruses	ssRNA,+ve sense, nonsegmented genome, enveloped	human — at least two	**rhinitis**
Orthomyxoviruses	ssRNA −ve sense segmented genome, enveloped		
Influenza A		three — human H_1N_1, H_2N_2, H_3N_2	rhinitis, **pharingitis, tracheobronchitis laryngotracheobronchitis**
Influenza B			**(croup)** bronchiolitis **pneumonia**
Paramxyoviruses	ssRNA,−ve sense nonsegmented genome, enveloped		
Parainfluenza		I,II,III,IV	rhinitis, **pharyngitis laryngotracheobronchitis (croup) bronchiolitis pneumonia**
Respiratory syncytial virus (RSV)		A and B sub-groups	rhinitis, pharyngitis laryngotracheobronchitis, **bronchiolitis, pneumonia**
Adenoviruses	dsDNA genome. nonenveloped	1,2,3,4,5,6,7, 14,21	rhinitis, pharyngitis, pneumonia

during infection selects new strains of virus produced by antigenic drift of virus surface receptor proteins. Within the rhinovirus group there are 102 serotypes associated with the common cold which presumably have evolved with antibody pressure. These different serotypes may coexist in the community giving rise to recurrent colds. With influenza A viruses antigenic drift allows the virus to evade the immune system giving rise to new epidemics every 2–3 years. In addition, influenza viruses are capable of high rates of recombination, during infection with different strains of virus, due to the segmented virus genome which allows reassortment of RNA segments during replication. Influenza A viruses infect a wide range of mammals and birds, both wild and domesticated, including pigs, horses, ducks and chickens, and therefore there is a large gene pool for reassortment. Typically with influenza A viruses this can lead to greater changes in the two surface glycoproteins leading to major epidemics and pandemics when a new antigenic strains arise. The different serotypes of influenza A are characterized based on these two surface glycoproteins the hemagglutinin (HA) and the neuraminidase (NA). There are a total of 13 different HAs known in animals of which three are found in human infections, and nine NAs of which two have been associated with human disease. It is believed that the close proximity of man with domesticated and agricultural animals, particularly in countries in the Far East, such as China, where the major pandemics of recent times have originated, allows for reassortment with animal influenza viruses. Influenza B viruses infect only humans and do not possess the variability seen with influenza A. Antigenic drift occurs with influenza B giving rise to minor epidemics typically in children each or every other year. The parainfluenza viruses have four serotypes of which types 1 and 2 generally alternate causing outbreaks of disease every other year and type 3 every year. Respiratory syncytial virus, typically associated with disease in babies under 2 years of age, causes outbreaks of disease every year. This virus is antigenically relatively homogenous but has been typed based on the surface G glycoprotein into two sub-groups A and B which appear to cocirculate in the community in varying proportions in different years.

The antigenic variability of many of these viruses has severely limited the development and use of vaccines against respiratory viruses. Combined vaccination against influenza A and B viruses is of value in the elderly and chronically sick and those at risk of heart complaints. However, influenza vaccines are only modestly effective and poor responses are seen particularly in the elderly. Antigenic variablility means that constant epidemiological surveillance is necessary and new vaccines have to be produced every 2–3 years, and when a new pandemic strain arises there is a delay before a new vaccine may be produced. Vaccination against respiratory syncytial virus with formalin inactivated virus was found to exacerbate the disease in young babies. Therefore, respiratory viruses are important agents for chemotherapy, particularly since highly conserved virus proteins may be targeted. However, the high specificity required for virus inhibitors and the diverse group of viruses involved mean that it is unlikely that one inhibitor will be active against all respiratory viruses, but that several inhibitors will be developed for specific virus groups. Ideally hand-in-hand with such developments would be required rapid early diagnostics to confirm which virus is involved with the disease syndrome. Significant progress has and is being made with virus diagnostics particularly with enzyme immunoassays (EIA) and with the polymerase chain reaction (PCR) technology. The acute nature of virus respiratory disease requires early treatment for maximum benefit to limit damage to the respiratory epithelium.

Research into chemotherapy of respiratory infections has concentrated mainly on three virus groups. The influenza A and B viruses have been the major focus because of the high morbidity and increased mortality associated with epidemic and pandemic years. The rhinoviruses which cause 50% of all colds are considered a second important target. Although the disease syndrome is generally mild, the economic cost due to loss of man hours is substantial. The third virus, respiratory syncytial virus, typically causes severe disease in young babies leading to death in about 1% of cases. The following section will discuss progress made in developing therapies against these virus infections.

4.2 Influenza: virus and disease

Typical uncomplicated A infection is a tracheobronchitis, with small airway involvement, where the main symptoms are headache, chills, and dry cough, which are rapidly followed by a characteristic high fever and aching joints. The fever generally peaks at 24 h and persists for 3–4 days, but in some cases a second transient rise occurs. Frequently respiratory symptoms, such as runny nose and coughing, may increase as the fever declines. Whilst most symptoms resolve by 7 days, the cough and general weakness may persist up to 3 weeks after infection. Influenza B produces similar symptoms but is generally milder with less pronounced fever and myalgia. However, with influenza A the severity of disease varies tremendously from asymptomatic infections to occasional cases of primary viral pneumonia where death may occur within 24–72 h of infection. In children influenza causes similar symptoms but higher fevers may lead to convulsions and there is a higher incidence of otitis media (middle ear infection) and of gastrointestinal manifestations such as vomiting and abdominal pain. Influenza-associated croup may be severe in young children. Classical influenza is therefore not a trivial disease, with epidemics and pandemics associated with significant increases in death, particularly in the elderly, but also in other age groups, including the very young. In the 1919 'Spanish' pandemic, deaths were estimated at 20 million.

Influenza A and B viruses are structurally similar but are distinguished antigenically by the reactivity of their internal nucleocapsid, the complement-fixing antigen. The structure of the influenza A virus is described below, indicating differences with the influenza B virus and is represented diagramatically in *Figure 4.1*. The genome of the influenza virus is segmented negative sense RNA (13 kD) consisting of eight RNA segments which code for a total of 10 proteins (11 proteins, influenza B), with the two smallest RNA segments (three smallest, influenza B) producing two transcripts each by differential splicing during

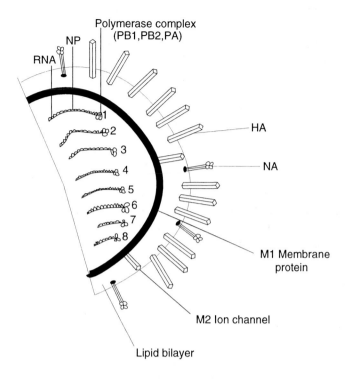

Figure 4.1: Influenza virus structure.

transcription. The function of these 10 proteins, 8 structural, that are present in the virus particle and 2 nonstructural, present only in the infected cell, are listed, where known, in *Table 4.2*.

During virus replication (see *Figure 4.2*), the HA spike recognizes *N*-acetyl-neuraminic acid (sialic acid) present terminally on glycoconjugates, as the receptor for cell attachment. After attachment the virus is invaginated into cellular endosomes where, under acidic conditions, protons enter the virus via the M2 ion channel (NB protein in influenza B), leading to a pH-induced conformational change in HA, where HA2 becomes accessible to induce fusion of the virus and cellular membranes, resulting in release of the ribonucleoprotein complexes (RNPs) into the cell. These RNPs are transported to the nucleus where primary virus transcription occurs, that is transcription of the vRNA by the polymerase, present in virus, into mRNA ready for translation. Transcription of influenza virus is unique in that the virus polymerase complex recognizes the cap structures on cellular mRNA, cleaves the cap structure plus 10–13 nucleotides and uses it as a primer for virus mRNA synthesis. The eight mRNA segments produced are translated and two messages spliced by the cell. Later, a switch to synthesis of non-capped full-length complementary RNA occurs mediated by the virus nucleoportein, from which

Table 4.2: Influenza virus gene products and function

Segment	Protein	Function
1	PB2	Part of virus RNA transcriptase complex. Cap-binding of host cell mRNA, ?endonuclease.
2	PB1	Part of virus RNA transcriptase complex. Catalyses nucleotide addition / RNA chain elongation ?endonuclease.
3	PA	Part of virus RNA transcriptase complex, function unknown.
4	HA	Surface glycoprotein, major antigenic determinant, binds cell receptor via sialic acid residues. Fusion with cell membrane at acid pH.
5	NP	Binds to RNA to form coiled ribonucleoprotein, involved with switch from virus mRNA to cRNA and in vRNA synthesis.
6	NA	Surface glycoprotein, antigenic determinant, neuraminidase activity involved with spread of virus.
7	M1	Major component of virus forming protein layer underneath lipid bilayer.
	M2	Integral membrane protein, ion channel, at acid pH protons enter virion to trigger conformational change in HA and fusion.
8	NS1	Nonstructural protein found in cell nucleus, nucleolus and cytoplasm involved with transport of virus mRNA to the nucleus.
	NS2	Nonstructural protein in cytoplasm and nucleus, function unknown.

vRNA will be produced for the progeny virus. Further mRNA (secondary transcription) will be transcribed by the newly formed RNPs and a total of 10 virus proteins produced. Accumulation of virus proteins in the cell membrane and alignment of RNP complexes below results in the budding of virus from the cell membrane.

4.3 Influenza: antiviral drugs

4.3.1 Amantadine/ rimantadine

Amantadine hydrochloride (Symmetrel™) and its close analog α-methyl-1-adamantanemethylamine hydrochloride (rimantadine, Flumadine™, Roflual™) (see *Figure 4.3*) were first reported to possess potent anti-influenza A activity in

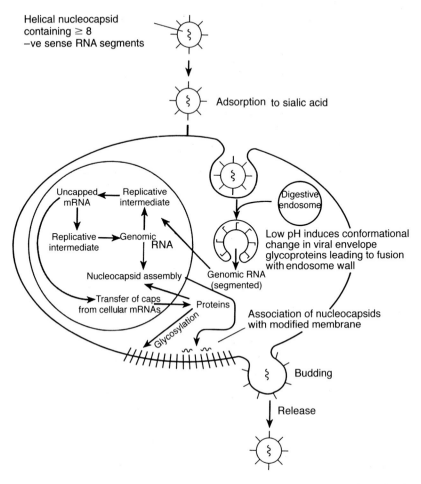

Helical nucleocapsid
containing ≥ 8
−ve sense RNA segments

Adsorption to sialic acid

Uncapped
mRNA

Replicative
intermediate

Digestive
endosome

Replicative
intermediate

Genomic
RNA

Low pH induces conformational
change in viral envelope
glycoproteins leading to fusion
with endosome wall

Nucleocapsid assembly

Genomic RNA
(segmented)

Transfer of caps
from cellular mRNAs

Proteins

Glycosylation

Association of nucleocapsids
with modified membrane

Budding

Release

Figure 4.2: Influenza virus replication. (Reproduced from Harper, D.R. (1998) *Molecular Virology.* 2nd Edn. BIOS Scientific Publishers, Oxford, in press.)

cell culture and in animal models (mouse and ferret) in 1964 [1] and 1965 [2], respectively. Their spectrum of activity is confined to influenza A strains only, with no significant activity against influenza B, or parainfluenza viruses or respiratory syncytial virus, despite early reports to the contrary. Even with influenza A, some of the early 1930 (H_1N_1) isolates were relatively insensitive although human isolates since the late 1940s including the H_1N_1, H_2N_2 and H_3N_2 serotypes are sensitive. In cell culture 50% inhibition of virus growth is seen at concentration around 0.05–1.0 μM (0.01–0.2 $\mu g\ ml^{-1}$) for both inhibitors, and *in vivo* at doses of 50–100 mg kg^{-1} day^{-1}.

Early studies showed that amantadine hydrochloride inhibited an early stage in the replication of human influenza strains, blocking uncoating and release of the virus genome into the cell. It was not until more than a decade later that the

molecular basis for the specific anti-influenza action of amantadine was elucidated. Initially recombination studies with an early resistant strain A/Bel/42
(H_1N_1) and an amantadine sensitive strain A/Japan/57 (H_2N_2) demonstrated that
resistance was linked to RNA segment 7 which codes for the M proteins. Further
studies revealed that it was the M2 protein which conferred resistance to amantadine and that four amino acids, residues 27, 30, 31 and 34 within a hydrophobic
transmembrane sequence were involved. Resistant mutants were cross-resistant to
rimantadine confirming that both compounds inhibit virus by the same mechanism. Subsequently it was demonstrated that the M2 protein of influenza A strains,
present as a homotetramer, forms an ion channel through the virus membrane.
Amantadine, by blocking the passage of protons through this M2 ion channel,
inhibits the pH-induced conformational change in HA required for the release of

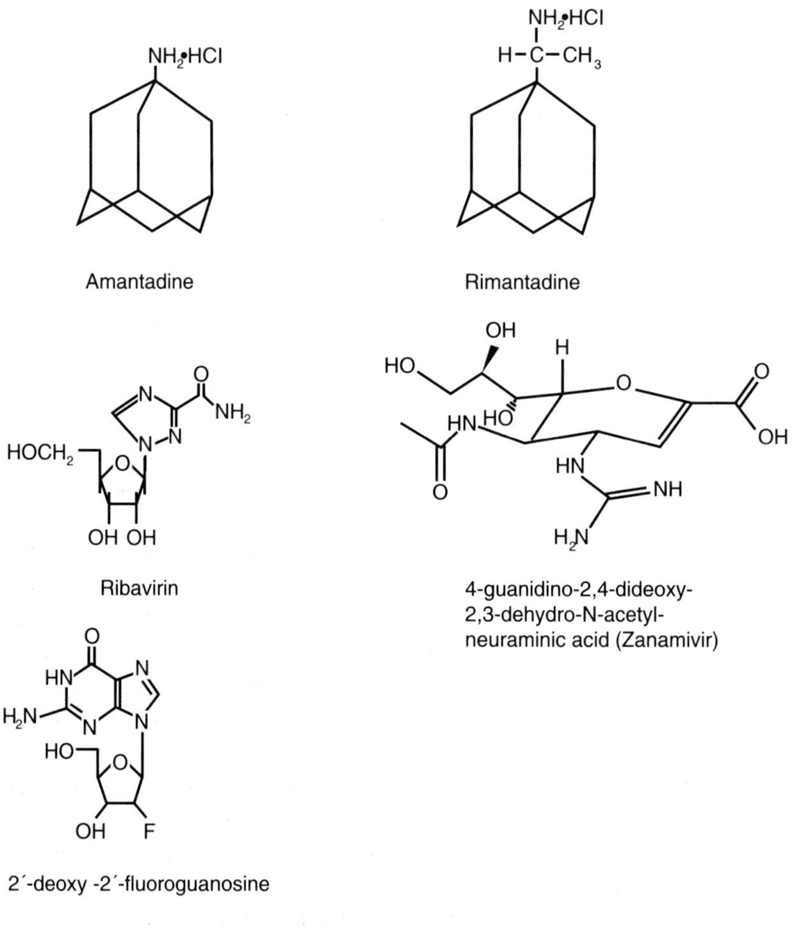

Figure 4.3: Structures of influenza inhibitors.

the RNP complexes into the cell. With one of the avian influenza strains, fowl plague virus, the pH optimum for the conformational change in HA is higher (pH 6) and this change occurs prior to virus budding through the cell membrane. Thus, although the mechanism of inhibition is the same, amantadine blocks a late stage in replication of fowl plague virus. This mechanism is mimicked in the anticholinergic activity of amantadine which blocks neuromuscular transmission by interacting with the ion channels of nicotinic acetylcholine receptors. In this context amantadine has also been used in the treatment of Parkinson's disease.

Preliminary clinical studies with any respiratory virus inhibitor are conducted under controled conditions by challenging volunteers intranasally with live virus and treating with inhibitor either before (prophylaxis) or after (therapy) infection. The earliest challenge trial with amantadine in 1964 showed a significant reduction in infection in volunteers pre-treated with amantadine. Further larger trials under natural epidemic conditions were therefore warranted. Early trials were designed to look at the prophylactic effect of amantadine, and the majority of trials demonstrated a beneficial effect with a 60–70% mean protective level. One prophylactic trial design which keeps most rigidly to normal environmental conditions involves family units where once one person in the family has been infected (index case) the remaining members of the family (contacts) were all treated with amantadine or placebo for 10 days. The first trial with this design was undertaken when A/England /10/67 (H_2N_2) was prevalent and there was a significant reduction in the incidence of serologically confirmed influenza in the contacts. Trials designed to establish if amantadine hydrochloride would be effective in treating influenza also demonstrated a beneficial effect provided the compound was administered within 48 h (preferably 24 h) after symptoms first appeared. These results were extremely encouraging, not only had amantadine proved to be the first drug that could prevent clinical influenza but also that it was possible to treat influenza effectively once symptoms had appeared. This later result indicated that virus is actively replicating during the disease syndrome and that replication is not largely complete by the time symptoms arise, as was originally assumed by many investigators.

Amantadine was registered for use against Asian influenza in 1966 at a recommended oral dose of 200 mg twice daily. When the Hong Kong influenza strain arose in 1968 and again when the H_1N_1 strains re-emerged in the 1970s, further trials were required to prove efficacy even though the drug was active in cell culture against these virus strains. Amantadine has not been used widely in the clinic, the main reasons seem to be lack of awareness that a treatment for influenza was available, and secondly, the CNS side-effects of amantadine including dizziness and insomnia. However, rimantadine has been shown to possess fewer side-effects than amantadine and to be equally effective in clinical studies at lower doses, 100 mg per dose twice a day. Rimantadine, although out of patent, was approved for use against influenza in the US in 1994.

More recent clinical studies have monitored clinical isolates for resistance development. In rimantadine trials resistant variants have been isolated in up to a third of treated patients, although beneficial effects on disease outcome were still seen. Resistant variants contained the same mutations as those seen in cell culture isolates. To date although amantadine has been used on a limited basis over 20 years and rimantadine has been widely used in the former USSR, no epidemics with resistant virus have occured. However, resistant viruses have been shown to have similar pathogenicity to wild-type virus in the ferret, and are transmissible and capable of causing disease in man. Possibly with the increased use of rimantadine transmission of resistant virus may become a problem unless the emergence of new influenza strains every few years limits the emergence of resistant virus.

4.3.2 Ribavirin

The nucleoside analog ribavirin (originally named virazole) (see *Figure 4.3*) was first synthesized in 1972 as part of a program to develop ribonucleoside analogs as potential broad-spectrum antiviral agents. Ribavirin was found *in vitro* to possess inhibitory activity against a number of both DNA and RNA viruses including influenza A and B, parainfluenza virus 1, respiratory syncytial virus and some of the exotic RNA viruses [3]. In cell culture ribavirin is less potent than amantadine with 50% inhibition seen at 10–30 µM (2.5–7.5 µg ml^{-1}). However, in the influenza mouse and ferret models significant inhibition was seen at doses from 36 to 150 mg kg^{-1} day^{-1} when administered orally or intraperitoneally.

In cells ribavirin is phosphorylated by cellular kinases to the 5´- monophosphate, diphosphate and triphosphate and probably exerts its antiviral effect by several mechanisms of action. The monophosphate blocks GMP biosynthesis by inhibiting the cellular enzyme inosine 5´-monophosphate dehydrogenase and thus affecting cellular nucleic acid synthesis by depletion of GTP pool levels. In addition, ribavirin triphosphate is an inhibitor of the influenza polymerase and blocks the cellular 5´-capping mechanism which is required for influenza replication, by inhibiting cellular guanylyl transferase activity. The specificity of ribavirin for virus inhibition is therefore low, since it probably exerts its main effects via cellular enzymes. This is supported by the finding that influenza and other viruses do not develop resistance to ribavirin *in vitro*.

In influenza challenge trials in volunteers in the US, ribavirin when administered orally at 600 mg day^{-1} produced at best marginal benefit either prophylactically or therapeutically against influenza A or B infections. A further challenge study with a higher dose, 1000 mg day^{-1}, against an influenza A strain produced only a slightly greater effect but at this dose ribavirin produced transient hematological abnomalities. Based on animal model data with influenza, this low efficacy would not have been predicted and probably reflects the rapid metabolism of ribavirin in man. Efforts were then directed to developing an apparatus to administer ribavirin directly to the respiratory tract as a small particle aerosol. In trials where ribavirin was administered as an aerosol for 12 h per day in the treatment of acute uncomplicated influenza A or B virus infections there was a significant reduction in symptoms and virus shedding, with no toxicological effects. Whilst this method of administration of ribavirin is only suitable for use in hospitalized cases of influenza, it has paved the way for more widespread use of ribavirin aerosols for the treatment of respiratory syncytial virus infections in babies (see 4.5.1). Nonetheless ribavirin has been lisensed for use in influenza infection in some countries. In addition, ribavirin has been evaluated clinically for the treatment of Lassa fever caused by an RNA virus of the *Arenaviridae* family. Ribavirin was effective when given orally or intravenously significantly reducing viraemia and mortality when administered at any time during illness but was most effective when given early.

4.3.3 Neuraminidase inhibitors : 4-guanidino-2, 4-dideoxy-2,3-dehydro-N-acetylneuraminic acid (GG167, zanamivir)

4-Guanidino-2,4-dideoxy-2,3-dehydro-*N*-acetylneuraminic acid, (zanamivir) (see *Figure 4.3*), described in 1993 [4], is the first inhibitor of influenza virus replication which has been designed based on the 3-dimensional structure of an influenza protein, the enzyme neuraminidase. The neuraminidase active site is highly conserved in all strains of influenza A and B sub-types. Several inhibitors of neuraminidase have previously been discovered either by random screening against the virus enzyme or by synthesizing substrate analogs, from which one of the most potent was 2-deoxy-2,3-dehydro-*N*-acetyl neuraminic acid (DANA). However, although DANA inhibited virus replication in cell culture it was not active *in vivo* casting doubt on the potential value of neuraminidase as a target for chemotherapy. Furthermore, DANA and other substrate analogs were not selective for the virus enzyme but caused significant inhibition of mammalian neuraminidases. Following the determination of the influenza A neuraminidase structure in 1982, a small biotechnology company (Biota) was set up to design inhibitors based on the enzyme structure with DANA bound within the active site. Using this structure, further substrate analogs were designed including zanamivir, where the guanidino group filled an empty pocket within the substrate binding region, leading to significant increases in potency and selectivity. Zanamivir was shown to be a selective high affinity competitive inhibitor of influenza neuraminidase for both influenza A and B strains with 50% inhibitory concentrations ranging from 0.64 to 7.9 nM, whereas mammalian neuraminidases are six orders of magnitude less sensitive. Against influenza A and B virus replication in cell culture zanamivir is extremely potent with 50% inhibitory activity ranging from 5 to 14 nM, but against clinical isolates the range was greater from 2 nM up to 16 µM. In both the mouse and ferret models zanamivir was efficacious when given by aerosol at low doses (0.01–0.4 mg kg^{-1} dose^{-1}) but not when administered systemically presumably due to the rapid clearance from the plasma. By aerosol, zanamivir was substantially more effective than amantadine or ribavirin administered by the same route. This is the first example of an influenza neuraminidase inhibitor with significant inhibitory activity *in vivo*.

Extensive studies have been undertaken to select for resistant viruses in cell culture. Resistant variants have been isolated, after prolonged exposure to the compound, with changes in the *HA* or *NA* genes or both. Some isolates with mutations in HA demonstrate drug dependence, producing increased growth in the presence of the compound. Changes in HA appear to be associated with reduced affinity for the sialic acid containing receptors allowing virus release from the cell in the absence of, or with reduced, NA activity. Drug dependence appears to result from increased adsorption of some of these slow binding viruses when the neuraminidase activity is blocked. Interestingly an HA variant was shown to be highly sensitive to zanamivir *in vivo* suggesting that the HA resistant phenotype may only be relevant *in vitro*. In the *NA* gene one significant mutation at residue 119 within the compound binding site is associated with resistance. However, these mutants show reduced neuraminidase stability and may not replicate as well *in vivo*.

Clinical studies are in progress. The first challenge study in volunteers with influenza A/Texas/91 (H_1N_1) was completed in 1994 and proved that zanamivir was efficacious in humans when administered as an aerosol at 16 mg per dose, six times daily. Both prophylactic administration, commencing 4 h before challenge, and therapy, commencing 26 h after challenge, were effective in reducing virus shedding and fever. Further trials under natural epidemic conditions have confirmed that zanamivir is effective in reducing symptoms in the treatment of influenza provided it is administered early after the onset of disease.

4.3.4 Polymerase inhibitors: 2´-deoxy-2´-fluororibosides

2´-Deoxy-2´-fluororibosides are a series of nucleoside analogs reported in 1993 [5] to possess potent inhibitory activity against influenza A and B strains. One of the most potent 2´-fluorodeoxyguanosine (FDG) has undergone more extensive studies. In cell culture anti-influenza potency varies with the cell line used to evaluate activity. The greatest potency was observed in human tracheal cultures and human nasal explants with efficacy (IC_{50} values) down to 0.1 µg ml^{-1} (0.33 µM) against influenza A and B strains with no toxicity at 100 µg ml^{-1}. In *in vivo* models the compound was effective systemically at 5–40 mg kg^{-1} day^{-1} and demonstrated greater potency than either amantadine or ribavirin.

In cell culture and *in vivo* FDG is rapidly phosphorylated to its 5´-triphosphate which acts as a selective, competitive inhibitor of the influenza polymerase/transcriptase, blocking elongation of the RNA chain during virus transcription. Partially resistant variants have been selected in cell culture showing a five-fold reduction in sensitivity. Analysis of the polymerase from a resistant variant demonstrated reduced affinity for the natural substrate indicating that the enzyme was partially crippled. This could explain the inability to push resistance further in cell culture. Sequencing of PB1 revealed one consistent sequence change observed in three separate resistant isolates at residue 492 which is highly conserved in all influenza strains.

Ribavirin is the only other polymerase inhibitor with activity *in vivo* against influenza. Interestingly, with both compounds, selection of resistant variants proved difficult or impossible suggesting that resistance may be less of a problem with inhibitors targeted to polymerase than with some other virus targets.

4.4 Respiratory syncytial virus: virus and disease

Human respiratory syncytial virus (RSV) is the major etiological agent associated with lower respiratory tract disease of young children worldwide, with yearly epidemics in children under 2 years of age. It is frequently associated with nosocomial infections in hospitalized children. After maternal antibodies have declined, at approximately 6 weeks of age, it is the leading cause of bronchiolitis (50% of all cases) and of pneumonia in infants.The incubation period is 4–5 days with initial symptoms of a common cold which spreads to the lower respiratory tract. Respiratory symptoms can develop rapidly with labored breathing, persistant cough, wheezing, emphysema and cyanosis in some cases, leading to death in up to 30% of cases, or after recovery within 7–12 days, to detectable reduced pulmonary dysfunction for months to years after infection. Immunity is short-lived so that repeat infections are possible, but generally milder, in adults. However, in immunocompromised adults and the elderly, RSV can be a significant cause of disease. Considerable efforts have gone into developing a vaccine for RSV infections but these have been hampered by the immunopathology associated with the disease. This means that there is a considerable need for chemotherapy or passive immunotherapy to limit the severity of the disease.

Respiratory syncytial virus is an enveloped virus containing two surface glycoproteins and a third transmembrane protein, with a nucleocapsid containing a nonsegmented genome which codes for a total of 10 proteins (see *Table 4.3*). Although classified in the Paramyxoviridae, RSV differs from the parainfluenza

Table 4.3: Respiratory syncytical virus gene products and function

Gene products	Function
G	Surface glycoprotein spike involved with attachment to cell receptor.
F	Surface glycoprotein spike. Proteolytically cleaved to produce disulfide linked F_1 and F_2. F_1 involved with fusion of virus envelope with host cell during virus entry. F_1 fusion of cell membranes produces syncytia formation.
M	Inner lining of virus envelope.
M2	Virus envelope, function unknown.
N	Nucleocapsid tightly complexed to the RNA genome.
L	Polymerase, component of ribonucleoprotein complex.
P	Component of polymerase complex.
SH	Surface of infected cell, membrane protein, function unknown.
NS1	Nonstructural protein, function unknown.
NS2	Nonstructural protein, function unknown.

viruses in that it lacks a neuraminidase and a hemagglutinin which are present in other paramyxoviruses in a combined form, the HN protein. The virus is relatively unstable and has not been studied as extensively as influenza.

During replication of the virus, the G glycoprotein surface spike binds to the cell receptor, and then the F glycoprotein surface spike or fusion protein, which is active at physiological pH, induces fusion with the cell membrane leading to penetration of the nucleocapsid. Like other negative-strand viruses RSV particles contain a virus polymerase that directs the copying of input vRNA into complementary mRNA (primary transcription) followed by synthesis of virus proteins. Subsequent progeny nucleocapsids will transcribe further mRNA (secondary transcription). The presence of gene start (nine conserved nucleotides) and stop (12–13 partially conserved nucleotides) signals results in the production of 10 discrete sub-genomic polyadenylated mRNAs which are translated into the 10 virus proteins. Synthesis of negative-strand RNA involves the synthesis of a complete positive sense copy of the vRNA by an anti-termination mechanism which causes the polymerase to ignore transcription signals. Progeny viruses mature by budding through regions of the plasma membrane that contain an accumulation of virus glycoprotein spikes.

4.5 Respiratory syncytial virus: antiviral drugs

4.5.1 Aerosol ribavirin

As indicated earlier ribavirin was first shown to posses anti-RSV activity in 1972 [3]. However, initial development concentrated on influenza prophylaxis and therapy culminating in the evidence that aerosol therapy was effective against influenza infections. This led to further studies with RSV infections in young babies.

In cell culture RSV replication is inhibited at 2.5–10 µg ml^{-1} (5–20 µM) concentrations of ribavirin. Subsequent studies in the cotton rat model in 1982, confirmed that ribavirin was efficacious when given, either systemically by intraperitoneal injection, or by aerosol 1 h after infection with RSV. This warranted further aerosol trials in man with RSV infection. Initially, ribavirin was evaluated in a challenge trial in adults who were treated for 12 h per day with aerosolized ribavirin. This resulted in significant reductions in systemic symptoms, fever and virus shedding, with no apparent adverse effects. This paved the way for further evaluation in infants with lower respiratory tract disease due to RSV. For initial studies in infants the small particle aerosol generator was used with an oxygen hood, or oxygen tent and continuous aerosol (20 h day^{-1}) was given for 3–6 days. Under these conditions ribavirin was shown to improve symptoms significantly and to reduce virus shedding. A second study where ribavirin was administered for 12 h per day was also efficacious and no toxicity was observed in either trial. Virus isolates taken over the course of therapy were shown to have no change in their sensitivity to the drug. Ribavirin has been approved for use in infants with severe RSV infections in the US and in several other countries. However, there are concerns over the cost of therapy with ribavirin aerosols, problems associated with continuous delivery due to precipitation of the compound, and the limited benefit afford by the inhibitor.

4.5.2 Immunotherapy—polyvalent hyperimmune globulin

The two surface spikes, the F and G glycoproteins are important in eliciting neutralizing antibodies. However, RSV appears to induce an imperfect immune response in humans in that reinfection is common and vaccination with formalin-inactivated virus was found to exacerbate the infection. Despite this there is evidence in animals (cotton rats) that neutralizing antibody protects against infection. Furthermore, in new-born infants, RSV neutralizing antibody titers of 1:300–400, correlate with reduced disease severity. Therefore, it was reasoned that immunoprophylaxis with human intravenous immuno-globulin (IVIG) may be beneficial to high risk babies, that is premature babies under 6 weeks, children with bronchopulmonary dysplasia or congenital heart disease particularly associated with pulmonary hypertension. Two small trials with IVIG (Gamimune-N™) were undertaken in the US in 1988, using three different doses (500, 600, 750 mg kg^{-1}) with 1-monthly infusions over the respiratory season (3–5 months). The peak RSV antibody titers achieved were not high 1:124 at most, probably too low to afford protection. However, there was a trend towards less severe RSV as measured by hospital days (8.8 + 5 days, treated: 12.8 + 7.6 days, controls) and the infusion was safe with no adverse reactions. These studies prompted the development of an RSV enriched immuno-globulin (RSVIG) for therapy, prepared with plasma taken from donors with high RSV antibody titers [6]. A larger trial with RSVIG (high dose 750 mg kg^{-1} or low dose 150 mg kg^{-1}) over 3 years with 249 premature babies < 6 months old was initiated in 1989. The high dose RSVIG was safe and effective in decreasing the incidence and severity of RSV infections compared to the low dose or placebo control. Follow-up of children over the subsequent respiratory season showed no evidence of exaggerated RSV pulmonary illness after RSVIG treatment. A population of high risk babies have been identified, that is premature babies born too early to have acquired maternal antibody (<32 weeks gestation) who are less than 9 months of age, and babies with chronic pulmonary disorders less than 18 months of age during the respiratory virus season. A dosage of 750 mg kg^{-1} delivered intravenously over 2 h at monthly intervals from November to March/April is recommended in the US to help protect against RSV disease. Further clinical studies with different formulations of RSVIG, which have included a detergent virus inactivation step in production, have confirmed the beneficial effects of passive immunization against RSV in preterm children. Respigam™ approved for use in the US in high risk babies, has confirmed the value of immunotherapy for RSV, but supplies of RSVIG are limited.

4.5.3 Immunotherapy—monoclonal antibodies to the fusion protein

The fusion protein spike has been shown to be the major target for the cross-protective immune response to RSV. Murine monoclonal antibodies (mAbs) raised to the fusion protein were shown to protect mice from infection with RSV measured as a reduction in mouse lung titer when the mAbs were inoculated intravenously 24 h before challenge with virus. For use in human therapy a murine monoclonal antibody has to be modified or humanized because of the problem with immune response to the mouse protein. For the RSV fusion mAb a reshaped human antibody was produced by taking the hypervariable complementarity determining regions (CDRs) from the murine antibody and transplanting them into a human monoclonal antibody of similar structure. The resulting engineered antibody was effective in protecting mice against challenge with a number of A and B strains either by the intraperitoneal or aerosol routes. Interestingly this antibody was extremely effective in reducing mouse lung virus titers when given as a single 25 µg dose intraperitoneally from 1 to 4 days after virus challenge [7]. In monkeys the half-life was 21–24 days after iv administration. This demonstrated the potential of this approach for treating RSV infections in man. Although this particular mAb was dissapointing in man, a second more avid binding mAb (Medi-493) has been reported from Phase III clinical trials to reduce RSV associated hospitalization in high risk babies.

A second similar approach only using Fabs, the antibody binding fragments of monoclonal antibodies, targeted to the fusion protein, are being developed in the US [8]. Scientists at NIAID have used combinatorial libraries that express Fab fragments, derived from human bone marrow or peripheral blood, on the surface of filamentous DNA bacteriophages. These libraries may be screened with antigen, in this case the fusion protein of RSV, to select Fabs of interest. In this way Fabs to the RSV fusion protein have been selected and shown to be highly effective in the prophylaxis and therapy of RSV infections in the mouse when delivered by aerosol. The half-life of Fabs in plasma is very short therefore parenteral administration is of no value but aerosol Fab fragments proved as effective as whole IgG molecules. Based on these studies Fabs or $F(ab)_2$ fragments administered directly to the lungs by small particle aerosol may be useful in the therapy of RSV infections.These approaches have significant advantages over immunotherapy with RSVIG in that much lower quantities of antibody (~10 000 fold less) are required via the aerosol route and, being engineered, large quantities may be produced in *E. coli* at significantly reduced cost. Human trials with RSV neutralizing monoclonal antibodies are in progress and, if they live up to expectations from *in vivo* studies, would probably replace therapy with RSV polyvalent hyperimmune globulin.

4.6 Rhinoviruses: viruses and disease

Rhinoviruses are the major causative agents of the upper respiratory tract infections known to everyone as the common cold. Typical symptoms are sneezing, nasal obstruction, nasal discharge and sore throat, frequently accompanied by headache, cough and malaise. Occasionally other symptoms may accompany a cold including lower respiratory tract involvement and in 10–20% of cases mild fever. Nasal discharge is the most typical sign of infection and may be quantified in clinical trials by weighing used handkerchiefs, which for a typical cold over 3–5 days, will be on average 8.5 g, but can be as high as 85 g. Common colds may predispose some people to secondary bacterial infections such as sinusitis, otitis media, and chronic bronchitis and in chidren may precipitate asthma attacks. Infections are most frequent in young children with up to 6–10 colds per year in pre-school children but by adulthood that has reduced to fewer than 2–5 per year per adult. Nevertheless the high morbidity results in a substantial loss of working days which has significant economic consequences.

Rhinovirus particles are roughly spherical nonenveloped particles which consist of just a protein coat which is icosahedral in symmetry and surrounds the virus genome, a single-stranded positive sense RNA molecule which is linked covalently to a small virus encoded protein VpG. The protein coat is made up of 60 copies each of four capsid proteins VP1–4 arranged around a five-fold axis, the pentamer, which forms 12 corners of the icosahedron. Picornaviruses, including rhinoviruses, under suitable conditions, form stable crystals, capable of producing high resolution diffraction patterns in an X-ray beam. The 3-dimensional structure of rhinovirus 1A (minor group) and 14 (major group) have been solved which has been of great value in understanding virus uncoating and assembly and in the design of inhibitors to block virus entry.

For 90% of rhinoviruses (the major receptor binding group) the cell receptor involved with attachment is the intercellular adhesion molecule (ICAM-1), which is normally involved with binding integrin to promote lymphocyte adhesion. For the remaining 10% of rhinoviruses (the minor receptor binding group) the receptor has not been identified. From the 3-dimensional structure of the virus a 12 Å by 12–15 Å wide, 25 Å deep depression, or 'canyon', has been identified at each pentagonal vertex which is the site of attachment for ICAM-1 (see *Figure 4.6*). Following attachment rhinoviruses enter cells by a process of endocytosis where the acid conditions of the vesicle lead to conformational changes in the virion capsid. This results in release of VP4 possibly through a channel at the center of the pentameric unit, and ultimately in release of the viral RNA genome into the cell cytoplasm where replication occurs. The positive sense RNA message is translated by the host cell translation machinery as a single open reading frame into one large polyprotein (*Table 4.4, Figure 4.4*). Two virus proteases, 2A and 3C, after self cleavage, cleave the capsid and nonstructural proteins by inter- and intramolecular cleavage of the polyprotein. Production of the 2A protease results in shutoff of cap-dependent mRNA translation by binding to the eIF-4F transcription factor. Rhinovirus mRNA translation will proceed in the absence of cellular cap structures by initiation at the cap-independent internal ribosomal entry site (IRES) at the 5′ end of the virus genome. One of the virus proteins synthesized is an RNA-dependent RNA polymerase which will catalyze the formation of negative sense intermediate and positive sense vRNA. Some of the vRNA will act as further

Table 4.4: Rhinovirus gene products and function

Gene products	Function
1A (VP1) 1B (VP2) 1C (VP3) 1D (VP4)	Virus capsid proteins, 60 copies of each per virion. VP1, 2 and 3 fold tightly to form a stable icosahedral shell with VP4 buried inside the viurs particle. Function to protect the virus RNA. VP1 involved with attachment to the cell receptor. Conformational changes lead to release of virus RNA into the cell.
2A	Protease cleavage of virus polyprotein. Inactivation of the cellular transcription fact eIF-4F leading to switch off of cell protein synthesis.
2B	Function unknown, possible determinant in host range.
2C	ATP-dependent helicase activity? Involved with virus RNA synthesis.
3A	Function unknown.
3B	VPg, covalently bound to the 5´ end of virus RNA via a tyrosine residue.
3C	Protease involved with cleavage of the virus polyprotein, and possible involvement with vRNA synthesis.
3D	RNA-dependent RNA polymerase.

message while some will be packaged into virus particles. Assembly of the capsid initiates with cleavage of the capsid precursor proteins to yield small 5S protomer complexes containing initially VP0 (a precursor of VP2 and 4), VP3 and VP1. These 5S protomers assemble into pentamers, 12 of which are required per virion to form the 60S sub-unit protein cell surrounding the virus RNA. Maturation of virus particles is complete when VP0 is cleaved to VP2 and 4. Mature virions are released by infection-mediated disintegration of the host cell.

4.7 Rhinoviruses: antiviral drugs

4.7.1 Capsid binding/canyon inhibitors

A number of structurally distinct inhibitors (*Figure 4.5*) of rhinovirus replication were discovered independently by several groups when randomly screening compounds against rhinovirus replication in cell culture in the late 1970s and early 1980s [9]. All these inhibitors have two common properties, firstly all are hydrophobic in nature, and secondly, all bind to the rhinovirus particle stabilizing the virion structure and blocking virus entry into the cell. These inhibitors are generally extremely potent, at least against some serotypes, inhibiting rhinovirus replication at nanomolar levels, but most show large variations in potency with different serotypes. The spectrum of activity of the different inhibitors varies with some showing relatively broad spectrum activity against most rhinoviruses and against

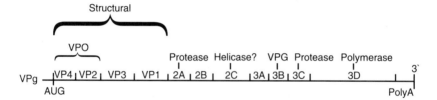

Figure 4.4: Rhinovirus genome structure.

some enteroviruses. Characteristically, in the presence of any of these inhibitors, resistant variants are easily isolated in cell culture. Cross-resistant variants confirmed that all these inhibitors have a similar target of inhibition.

At the time of discovery of the first inhibitors nothing was known about the site of binding on the virion. It was not until 1985 that the atomic structure of a human rhinovirus was first resolved and then it became possible to study compound binding by attempting to cocrystallize compounds bound to virus. In 1986, the structure of one of the inhibitors, disoxaril (Win51711) bound to rhinovirus 14 was solved (see *Figure 4.6*). This compound was found to bind in a hydrophobic pocket

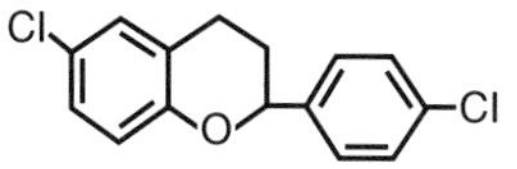

Dichloroflavan
(BW683)

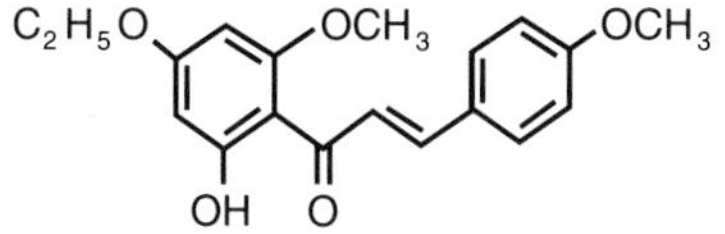

Ro09-0415
(chalcone)

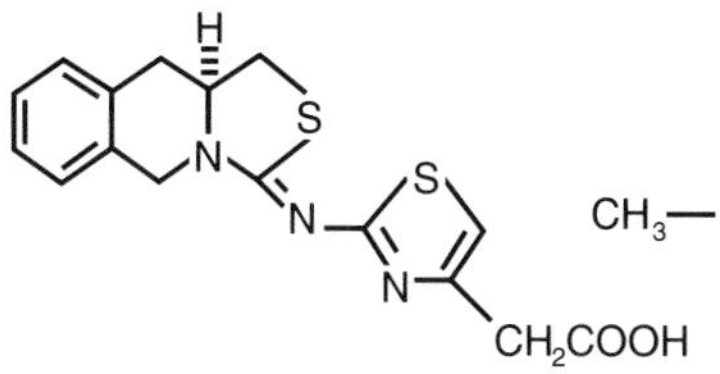

44,081R.P.

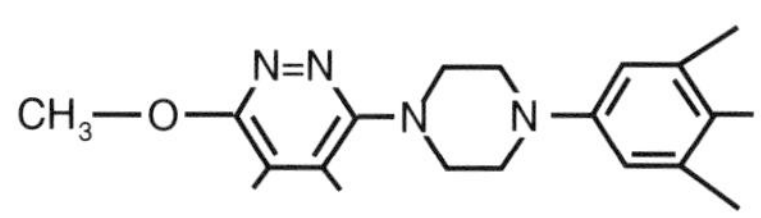

R61837
(Pirodavir)

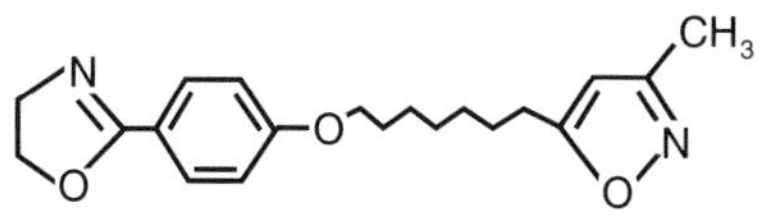

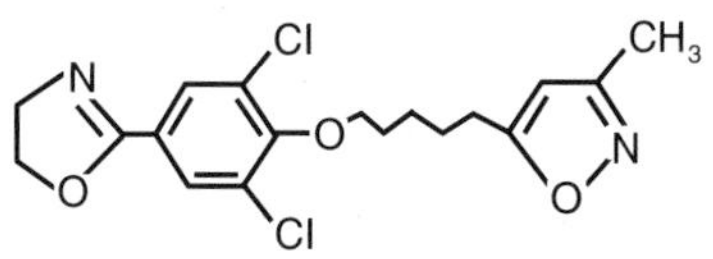

Figure 4.5: Structures of rhinovirus capsid binding agents.

inside VP1 beneath the floor of the canyon receptor binding region. Since there are 60 copies of VP1 per virion there must be 60 compound-binding sites per virion. Disoxaril blocks attachment of all the major receptor group viruses, whilst, with the minor group viruses it does not block attachment but prevents uncoating. Thus, binding to the hydrophobic pocket may block either attachment or uncoating. With rhinovirus 14, a major receptor group virus, binding resulted in a 5 Å shift in the position of the pocket resulting in changes to the floor of the canyon which blocks attachment to ICAM-1. With rhinovirus 1A, a minor receptor group virus, the binding pocket is much shorter than rhinovirus 14 and no conformational change was observed. Therefore conformational changes may be required to block attachment but not uncoating. A second feature was observed following drug binding, which was the apparent increased occupancy of a divalent cation at the vertex of each pentamer. It has been hypothesized that this may block release of VP4 which is present under the pentamer and as a result blocks uncoating. In addition, rhinovirus 1A was found to bind a cofactor, possibly a lipid in the drug binding pocket which was displaced by the inhibitor binding. Inhibitors may also bind in opposite orientations within the pocket highlighting the need for crystallographic data. Resistant variants to disoxaril were isolated and mutations were mapped to residues 188 and 199 in VP1, within the binding pocket. These mutations lead to

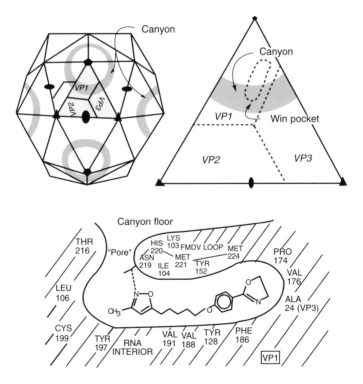

Figure 4.6: Rhinovirus capsid structure showing position of canyon, compound binding pocket and disoxaril bound into the pocket (Reproduced from International Antiviral News 1 (4), by permission of International Medical Press).

high level resistance and reduced drug binding. Mutants with lower resistance mapped to numerous sites outside the binding pocket and may block conformational shifts required for compound binding. Based on the structural data from rhinovirus 14 and 1A the inhibitor Win 54954, capable of binding more tightly than disoxaril to both viruses, has been designed.

There is no suitable animal model for human rhinoviruses, however some of the compounds with broader spectra of activity have been tested against related enteroviruses. For example, Win54954 was found to be orally available and to protect mice from developing paralysis at daily doses of 1.2–100 mg kg^{-1}day^{-1} when administered intraperitoneally to suckling mice previously infected with coxsackie virus A-9 or echovirus-9.

Many of the capsid binder inhibitors have been evaluated in rhinovirus challenge studies in volunteers, using a rhinovirus serotype which has been shown to be highly sensitive to the inhibitor in cell culture. In these studies a double-blind comparison of inhibitor and placebo is undertaken where a wide range of cold symptoms are scored depending on severity, along with measuring nasal mucous discharge weight and body temperature. Evaluation of some of the earlier capsid binders were disappointing. Neither dichloroflavan nor a phosphate prodrug of Ro09-0415 were effective when administered orally, even though plasma levels were in excess of the *in vitro* IC$_{50}$ values. However, neither compound was detectable in nasal secretions indicating that possibly neither compound reached the site of virus replication, the nasal epithelium. An alternative strategy was to administer these inhibitors by intranasal delivery. Again, dichloroflavan, Ro09-0410 and 44,081RP offered no protection against rhinovirus infection suggesting that possibly the compounds were not present in sufficient quantities due to rapid cilliary clearance. Analysis of virus from the nasal cavity of patients treated with Ro09-0415, however, demonstrated the presence of resistant virus which may account for the lack of efficacy. Desite the clinical failure of these early compounds some success was achieved with later inhibitors developed by Jansen pharmaceuticals. The most effective was Pirodavir formulated as a nasal spray at 5 mg ml^{-1} in 100 mg ml^{-1} hydroxypropyl-β-cyclodextrin. Cold symptoms and virus shedding were significantly reduced when the compound was given six times a day for 5 days. Little effect on symptoms was observed if dosing was reduced to three times a day although there was a significant reduction in virus shedding. Measurement of drug levels in nasal wipes and pharangeal swabs revealed that even with cyclodextrin formulations, designed to increase compound availability, drug only remained at significant levels for 30 min after dosing. This implies that slow release formulations are required to maintain significant drug levels in the nose for maximum effectiveness.

The most potent Sterling Winthrop inhibitor (Win54954) designed partly based on the structure of the drug binding pocket has also been evaluated in man. The compound was administered orally at 600 mg dose^{-1} three times daily commencing 24 h before challenge. Again results were disappointing with no reduction in cold symptoms and low compound levels in nasal secretions despite the presence of significant plasma levels. In contrast, in a similar intranasal challenge trial with coxsackie A21 there was a significant reduction in cold symptoms with orally administered compound. This is difficult to explain since both viruses have similar sensitivity to the inhibitor. Therefore, despite considerable progress made in understanding how these inhibitors function structurally there is still further work required to develop an inhibitor with potent activity in man. Structural studies have revealed that the drug binding pocket is unique for each rhinovirus and, therefore, further structural data is required from other rhinoviruses before attempts may be made to design a 'consensus' pocket for development of a broad spectrum drug. In addition, at least with strongly hydrophobic inhibitors, further improvements on drug formulations are required to achieve significant sustained drug levels within the nasal epithelium.

4.7.2 Interferon

Interferon was discovered in 1957 after incubation of chick chorioallantoic membrane with heat inactivated influenza virus. Following on from this initial observation, RNA viruses, in general, were found to be good inducers of interferon, and respiratory infections were considered to be good candidates for local treatment with interferon applied to the nasopharynx. However, it was several years later before sufficient quantities of interferon, produced from human leukocytes obtained from a human blood banks, were available for such studies. This first rhinovirus challenge study, carried out at the MRC Common Cold Unit using relatively crude human leukocyte interferon, proved that intranasally administered interferon could prevent infection with rhinovirus. By this time it was realized that interferon was in fact a family of interferons with three main types, IFN-α and IFN-β produced in response to virus infections in leukocyte and fibroblasts respectively, and IFN-γ produced in response to mitogens on unstimulated lymphoid cells. Large scale production and purification of interferon was achieved from lymphoblastoid (IFN-α) and fibroblastic human cell lines (IFN-β). Further significant progress toward large scale production of interferons was made when the different interferons were cloned and expressed in bacterial systems. Recombinant interferons (rIFN) have allowed more extensive evaluation to be made against rhinovirus infection [10]. Further prophylactic challenge studies with purified interferon from human leucocytes, human lympblastoid cells and with recombinant interferons (rIFN- 2α: IFN-αA) have clearly shown protection against experimental colds induced by a number of different rhinovirus serotypes. The level of protection was dose related but was also dependent on the duration of pretreatment before challenge. From these studies it may be concluded that short duration, high dose interferon 22–46 MU day^{-1} completely blocks infection with no detectable immunological response to infection. Lower doses 10 MU day^{-1} allow sub-clinical infections to occur with antibody responses. However, low doses (2 MU day^{-1}) were only protective if administered for a week before infection. Interestingly, interferons persist in the cells of the nasal mucosa for long periods, up to 18 h, allowing once-a-day treatments. The mode of administration, nasal drops or nasal sprays appeared to effect efficacy, and coadministration of anti-histamines improved efficacy of low dose interferon. In prophylactic challenge studies with coronavirus, the other important group of common cold viruses, interferon demonstrated beneficial effects. In contrast, interferon therapy, after rhinovirus challenge, produced only modest clinical benefit with high doses of 27 MU day^{-1} where significant reductions in virus shedding were observed.

Following on from the successes of the prophylactic challenge studies, trials were designed to evaluate prophylactic interferon in natural respiratory virus infections. Such trials have been conducted in two ways, firstly administering interferon daily over several weeks during the respiratory season, and secondly short-term post-exposure in family-based studies. In the long-term studies rIFN-α-2b was effective at 2-3 MU day^{-1} in the prevention of rhinovirus infections. However, daily administration for more than 2 weeks was associated with local toxicity, including nasal stuffiness, irritation, and blood-tinged mucus. Long-term prophylaxis with interferon in healthy patients would be unacceptable. In post-exposure prophylactic studies, again rIFN-α was protective, but only at relatively high doses 5 MU day^{-1}. In these studies protection was not afforded to other respiratory viruses including influenza, parainfluenza and coronavirus. Finally, treatment of established natural colds even using high doses 10–20 MU day^{-1} did not reduce symptoms or the duration of the colds and was associated with local side effects. Overall the beneficial prophylactic effects of IFN-α are severely compromised by the local side-effects. Further studies with the other interferon sub-types have been disappointing. With r-IFN-β local toxicity was reduced but so was efficacy, and with rIFN-γ at 6 MU day^{-1} there was no prophylactic effect and significant toxicity. Other IFN-α forms are being evaluated, but only if one is found with a significantly improved therapeutic ratio will prophylactic interferon for the prevention of the common cold be possible.

4.8 Future targets and therapies

Although significant progress has been achieved in developing specific inhibitors of the different respiratory viruses, in clinical terms the success is limited. In the future, with further application of molecular techniques and structural studies to some of the virus target proteins, rapid progress towards more effective clinical candidates should be possible.

The influenza inhibitors designed to block neuraminidase hold the most promise for the immediate future for control of influenza. However, the surface proteins of influenza are able to accommodate large numbers of mutations, and, although the active site of the neuraminidase is conserved suggesting that there may be limits on resistance development in the clinic with this class of inhibitor. Similar drug design techniques are also being applied to the hemagglutinin receptor but to date no potent inhibitors have been described. An important target for chemotherapeutic intervention is influenza transcription, where several functions unique to the virus are essential, such as cap-binding, endonuclease and transcriptase activities. As demonstrated with ribavirin and 2´-fluorodeoxyguanosine there may be constraints on resistance development to transcriptase inhibitors. Recently the first specific inhibitor of the endonuclease of influenza virus, a dioxobutanoic acid, has been described, which blocks influenza replication in cell culture. Antisense oligonucleotides have also been shown to block influenza transcription. The three proteins of the influenza transcriptase complex will only function as a complex, and on cloning into different expression systems produce low levels of protein. Therefore structural studies are not feasible at present. Other candidates for structural studies are the two nonstructural proteins, NS1 and NS2. Studies with NS1 have demonstrated that this protein possesses an RNA binding domain and is involved with RNA transport. The protein has been expressed to high level in *E. coli* and purified for structural studies.

The most promising therapies at present for RSV are the immunotherapies particularly the monoclonal antibodies to the fusion protein. Possibly combination therapy with ribavirin plus immunotherapy will be most advantageous in the therapy of severe disease. RSV has not been studied as extensively as influenza and less is known about RSV transcription. However, important advances are being made in developing an *in vitro* replication assay for RSV which should be valuable for chemotherapeutic studies in the future.

Further design of broad spectrum capsid binders against the different serotypes of rhinoviruses will require additional structural data from other rhinoviruses and the construction of a consensus pocket. This approach demands considerable resources and may require the development of combinations of inhibitors to overcome problems of spectrum and resistance, since one inhibitor is unlikely to bind optimally to a range of pocket configurations. A second interesting virus surface target is the virus receptor, recently identified to bind to ICAM-1, for the major group rhinoviruses. A soluble form of ICAM-1 is able to inhibit the cytopathic effect induced by the major group binders in susceptible cells. Receptor analogs may have potential in blocking virus attachment but again resistance may be a problem. For rhinoviruses as well, transcription is an important target with at least two essential enzymes the RNA-dependent RNA transcriptase (protein 3D) and the associated ATP-helicase (protein 2C) involved. The target with the most immediate potential for rhinovirus chemotherapy is the cysteine protease 3C for which the X-ray structure has recently be solved. This protein is highly conserved in all picornaviruses and therefore designed inhibitors should have a broad spectrum of activity with hopefully less potential for resistance development. Further, the 3C protein may play a role in vRNA synthesis in addition to protease cleavage.

In conclusion, significant progress is being made on understanding the structure and function of several essential proteins involved with the replication of the different respiratory viruses. Some of these areas of research should culminate in the development of new potent drugs for the clinic.

References

1. Davies, W.L., Grunert, R.F., Haff, J.W., McGahen, J.W., Neumayer, E.M., Paulshock, M., Watts, J.C., Wood, T.R., Hermann, E.C. and Hoffman, C.E. (1964) *Science*, **144**, 862.

2. Tsundo, A., Maassab, H.F., Cochran, K.W. and Eveland, W.C. (1965) *Antimicrobial Agents and Chemother.,* **13**, 139.

3. Sidwell, R.W., Huffman, J.H., Khare, G.P., Allen L.B., Witkowski, J.T. and Robins, R.K. (1972) *Science*, **177**, 705.

4. Von Itzstein, M., Wu, W-Y., Kok, G.G., Pegg, M.S., Dyason, J.C., Jin, B., Phan, T.V., Smythe, M.L., White, H.F., Oliver, S.W., Colman, P.M., Varghese, J.N., Ryan, D.M., Woods, J.M., Bethell, R.C., Hotham, V.J., Cameron, J.M. and Penn, C.R. (1993) *Nature (London)* **363**, 418.

5. Tuttle, J.V., Tisdale, M. and Krenitsky, T.A. (1993) *J. Med. Chem.* **36**, 119.

6. Groothius, J.R. (1994) *Pediatric Infect. Dis. J.,* **13**, 454.

7. Taylor, G., Furze, J., Tempest, P.R., Bremner, P., Carr, F.J. and Harris, W.J. (1991). *Lancet*, **337**, 1411.

8. Crowe, J.E., Murphy, B.R., Chanock, R.M., Williamson, R.A., Barbas III, C.F. and Burton, D.R. (1994) *Proc. Natl Acad. Sci.USA,* **91**, 1386.

9. McKinlay, M.A., Pevear, D.C. and Rossmann. M.G. (1992) *Ann. Rev. Microbiol.,* **46**, 635.

10. Hayden, F.G. (1988) in *Clinical Aspects of Interferons,* (M. Revel, ed.) Kluwer Academic Publishers, Boston, p. 3.

Further reading

R.M. Krug *et al.* (1989) *The Influenza Viruses* (R.M. Krug, ed.). Plenum Press, New York.

C.R. Pringle *et al.* (1991) *The Paramyxoviruses* (D.W. Kingsbury, ed.). Plenum Press, New York.

Chapter 5

Chemotherapy of hepatitis virus infections

5.1 Introduction: diversity of viruses associated with hepatitis (A,B,C,D,E)

The various agents responsible for viral hepatitis collectively impose a huge infectious burden on mankind and effective control of them would represent a major advance in human health care. In this chapter only those viruses for which the liver is the principal or only site of replication will be discussed and so viruses such as yellow fever virus, for which the liver is but one of a variety of target tissues, will not be included. As will be seen, the diverse group of viruses which cause viral hepatitis share a number of common features which presumably arose as adaptations to their particular ecological niche. One property which they all share is that of being extremely difficult to culture *in vitro* and replication can only be observed after extensive adaptation to tissue culture, or occurs at such low frequency or level as to be of little use for virological research. Mature hepatocytes rapidly lose many of their differentiation markers when grown *in vitro*, so that even primary hepatocytes in culture are significantly different from *in vivo* tissue, and it would appear that essential factors required for successful infection by the hepatotrophic viruses are amongst those which disappear first. This has been a major obstacle to the identification and study of the hepatotrophic viruses, as emphasized by the fact that an important member of the group, hepatitis C virus, was only identified as recently as 1989 and reports of further potential human hepatotrophic viruses have just appeared at the time of writing. These viruses have been identified using sophisticated methods of nucleic acid amplification and cloning which do not rely on the ability to culture the agents *in vitro*.

The hepatotrophic viruses are referred to by an alphabetical nomenclature system which has gradually evolved over the years. The designation of letters to viruses does not necessarily relate to the chronology of their discovery. The letters A and B were first used to distinguish hepatitis which could be transmitted orally in volunteers (A) from that which could not (B) and as diagnostic reagents became available they were used to signify the specific viral agents hepatitis A virus (HAV) and hepatitis B virus (HBV). HAV was later shown to be a member of the picornavirus family, albeit an unusual one, whereas HBV was identified as belonging to a previously unknown virus family, now known as the Hepadnaviridae. However, following the development of serological diagnostic tests for these two viruses, it soon became apparent that there were cases of hepatitis which could not be ascribed to HAV or HBV and these were referred to as nonA nonB (NANB) hepatitis. Furthermore, epidemiological studies showed that there were at least two further agents with distinct transmission characteristics. The major causative agent for enterically transmitted NANB hepatitis was identified as a calicivirus in the mid-1980s and termed hepatitis E virus (HEV); the E being derived from (E)nterically transmitted. Later, after a number of false alarms, the causative agent of NANB transfusion associated hepatitis was finally identified in 1989 by the cloning of cDNA prepared from the serum of an experimentally infected chimpanzee and was termed hepatitis C virus (HCV). The genome organization of HCV clearly placed it in the family Flaviviridae although it had little sequence homology to known members of that family. Hepatitis delta virus (HDV) is unique among animal viruses. It has a covalently closed single-stranded RNA genome, reminiscent of the plant viroids. It can be considered a satellite virus of HBV since it encodes no coat protein of its own and requires HBV envelope protein for encapsidation. It is named after the delta antigen which was found to be present in the nuclei of hepatocytes coinfected with the two viruses. More hepatotrophic viruses undoubtedly remain to be discovered; in fact, as mentioned above, there have been recent reports of new agents identified from tamarin marmosets infected with human samples or directly from human serum. The name hepatitis G virus (HGV) has been proposed for these new agents which also belong to the flavivirus family and are distantly related to HCV.

The hepatotrophic viruses are a taxonomically diverse group of agents as can been seen from their properties and classification as shown in *Table 5.1*. All but HBV have RNA genomes but belong to several different virus families. HBV has a small, circular, incomplete double-stranded DNA genome but replicates via an RNA intermediate using a polymerase with reverse transcriptase activity.

The viruses can be grouped according to biological properties which are related to the routes of transmission they have adopted and the nature of the infections they cause. Hepatitis A and E viruses are feco-orally transmitted and can cause large scale outbreaks due to contamination of water or foodstuffs when appropriate hygiene measures are lacking; for example, an outbreak of hepatitis A in China the 1980s resulted in the hospitalization of 600 000 patients and was traced to the consumption of contaminated clams. The feco-orally transmitted viruses, HAV and HEV, typically cause acute infections which are usually resolved and eliminated by host immune mechanisms over a period of a few weeks.

Hepatitis B, C and D viruses, however, are transmitted parenterally by direct blood contact and there is probably a functional linkage between this mode of transmission and the observation that these viruses are frequently associated with long-term chronic infections. HDV is rather different from the others in that it is dependent on coinfection with HBV in order to produce virus particles since it relies on the coat protein of HBV for encapsidation. Its transmission properties, therefore, are similar to those of HBV.

Table 5.1: Hepatotrophic viruses

Virus	Family	Genome characteristics	Genome size	Particle characteristic	Disease characteristics
Hepatitis A virus (HAV)	*Picornaviridae*	Nonsegmented +ve sense single-stranded RNA	7.5 Kb	Nonenveloped isometric	Acute, self limited
Hepatitis B virus (HBV)	*Hepadnaviridae*	Circular incomplete double-stranded DNA	3.2 Kb	Lipid envelope isometric core	Mostly acute, self limited in adults Mostly chronic persistent in infants
Hepatitis C virus (HCV)	*Flaviviridae*	Nonsegmented +ve sense single-stranded RNA	9.6 Kb	Lipid envelope isometric core?	Mostly chronic persistent irrespective of age when infected
Hepatitis Delta virus (HDV)	?	Circular single-stranded RNA	1.7 Kb	Lipid envelope HBV origin Nucleoprotein core with delta antigen	May exacerbate HBV pathology
Hepatitis E virus (HEV)	*Caliciviridae?*	Nonsegmented +ve sense single-stranded RNA	7.5 Kb	Nonenveloped isometric	Acute, self limited Often fatal in pregnant women
Hepatitis G virus (HGV)	*Flaviviridae*	Nonsegmented +ve sense single-stranded RNA	9.5 Kb	?	?

With most, and possibly all, of the hepatotrophic viruses infection of hepatocytes may not directly result in overt cytopathic effects on the cells. In fact, the
obvious symptoms of acute hepatitis often appear to be the result of destruction of
virus-infected cells by host immune mechanisms. Consequently, in acute, resolving infections the clinical evidence of disease occurs at the end stage of the process
when the host response is in the process of clearing infection. It is therefore unlikely to be greatly influenced by the administration of antiviral drugs. Therapeutic
intervention is of much greater potential relevance in the treatment of chronic
hepatitis since, although the short-term consequences of such infections may not
even be particularly severe, the long-term sequalae of chronic active hepatitis, cirrhosis and hepatocellular carcinoma are of major importance.

5.2 Likely impact of prophylaxis (vaccines, passive immunity)

As with all infectious agents, the use of effective vaccines, and hence prevention
of disease, is preferable to therapeutic intervention. However, vaccine development
has been slow for the hepatotrophic viruses, largely because of the innate problems
associated with the difficulties experienced in cultivating them. However, there are
now effective vaccines against HBV (and hence also HDV) and HAV.

The 'high tech' version of the HBV vaccine, which is used in the developed
world, is produced in yeast by recombinant DNA techniques. The vaccine consists
of purified s, or surface, antigen protein (HBsAg) of HBV, which has the innate
property of self assembly, together with host lipid components, into spherical and
rod like particles. The HBsAg is the major component of the outer lipid membrane
of both the mature virus or Dane particle (42 nm) and the HBsAg particles (22 nm)
and tubules found in large amounts in the sera of HBV carriers. It contains a major
group specific determinant which can elicit protective immune responses but lacks
some antigenic determinants found on the l and m proteins which are also components of the virus outer membrane. It was the first vaccine to be produced by
recombinant gene expression and its development represented a technological
triumph. However, the majority of the HBV vaccine used in the world today is produced by inactivation of viral material derived from the plasma of chronically
infected donors. Despite the obvious disadvantages of this source of antigen for
vaccine production, it does have the advantage that, although the major component
is HBsAg, it also contains the full range of HBV antigens and is highly immunogenic. Approximately 5–10% of recipients of the recombinant surface antigen
vaccine respond poorly due to incompatibility between their MHC protein
complement and the limited number of helper T-cell epitopes present in the molecule. There is, therefore a continuing need to develop new HBV vaccines which
are cheaper to produce and which include a wider range of viral antigens capable
of inducing good immunity in all vaccinees. Another concern stems from the identification of antigenically variant viruses which may be able to break vaccine
induced immunity. Whether vaccines which include these mutant antigens will
need to be developed is unclear at present.

Although the development and efficient use of HBV vaccines should eventually have a significant influence on the global situation, providing that these are administered effectively, there remains the problem of the vast number of chronically infected people (ca. 350 000 000) who form a huge reservoir of infectious virus and who are very likely to develop fatal liver disease. It is possible that vaccines may be beneficial when used therapeutically to stimulate a dormant immune response in chronically infected patients. Several groups are exploring this possibility using a variety of antigens ranging from conventional vaccine to synthetic peptide vaccines designed to stimulate specific cytotoxic T-cell responses.

Vaccines for HAV have also been developed and lisensed in the past few years. The antigen consists of formaldehyde inactivated tissue culture grown virus and is thus a conventional killed vaccine. The delay in producing and marketing this vaccine was in large part due to the low yield and slow growth cycle of the virus. The problem of producing significant amounts of virus for vaccine production were somewhat alleviated by the high immunogenicity of the antigen which ensures an effective immune response from a small amount of vaccine. Although the vaccine is safe and effective, its expense prohibits extensive use in any but the wealthiest countries, where it is least required.

Vaccines for the other hepatotrophic viruses are very much at the research and development stage. Production of HEV capsid protein by recombinant DNA technology is a potential route towards vaccine production which is being actively pursued. The extreme sequence, and hence assumed antigenic, diversity displayed by HCV does not auger well for the rapid development of vaccines for this virus but the prophylactic potential of expressed proteins is being studied.

In addition to vaccine development, passive immunization using serum immune globulins or monoclonal antibodies has played a role in approaches to combat viral hepatitis. Human immune globulin has been used for some years to protect travelers from areas nonendemic for HAV when visiting endemic areas. Although effective over a limited period, this procedure is likely to be replaced by vaccination, as this is now readily available. It does, however, provide the advantage of conferring instant protection against infection and disease.

Passive immunization plays an important role in the prevention of reinfection of new organs following liver transplantation in HBV positive patients and accounts for a high proportion of the total costs of the operation. It has also been claimed that passive immunization with relatively small amounts of anti-HBV monoclonal antibody can induce a curative response.

In conclusion, effective prophylactic vaccines exist for HAV and HBV although improvements need to be made to improve efficacy, in the case of HBV, and of reducing the cost for both before they will have a significant effect on the global burden of these two viruses. HDV control parallels that of HBV, since they share the same coat protein. A credible vaccine target molecule has been identified for HEV but, even if effective, production costs are likely to prohibit its extensive use in areas where the virus is a problem. With HCV it is difficult to see at present how an effective vaccine could be developed because of the high sequence diversity displayed by the virus, which is predicted to correlate with high antigenic variation, and also the apparent lack of protective immunity as evidenced by the failure of previous exposure to the virus to protect against reinfection in chimpanzees.

5.3 Chronic viral hepatitis: the main target for antivirals

5.3.1 Hepatitis B virus: structure and replication

HBV is the type member of the family Hepadnaviridae, which includes a number of viruses that infect mammalian or avian hosts. These viruses resemble the retroviruses in that during replication the genomic sequence is shuttled from RNA to DNA using a virally encoded reverse transcriptase, but differs from them in the timing of these events during the infectious cycle. In the Retroviridae the genome within the virus particle is RNA which is transcribed into DNA in the infected cell and then integrated into the host chromosomal DNA. In contrast, the hepadnavirus particle contains a circular DNA genome which consists of a complete negative strand and an incomplete positive strand and is thus only partially double-stranded. Synthesis of the positive strand is completed in the newly infected cell and the genome is converted into a covalently closed double-stranded circular structure which is transcribed by host cell DNA-dependent RNA polymerase into mRNAs and pregenomic viral RNA. This latter is packaged in core particles, along with the polymerase, and is there reverse transcribed into DNA. The replication cycle of the virus, therefore does not require integration into the host DNA.

HBV has a remarkably small genome consisting of only 3.2 Kb. However, this limited amount of sequence potential is utilized very efficiently since there are no untranslated regions and most of the genome codes for proteins in more than one reading frame. There are four main open reading frames, as shown in *Figure 5.1*, which are translated to produce a total of seven virus specific proteins (*Table 5.2*). The two ORFs which code for the structural proteins of the virus are translated as a series of nested products dependant on the precise transcription start sites used in the production of their messenger RNAs.

The nucleocapsid of the virus is built from the core protein, which is translated from the full length, pregenomic RNA transcript. It readily self assembles within the cell into icosohedral core particles containing pregenomic RNA and polymerase. These then acquire lipid envelopes containing the surface proteins and so become mature virus particles (*Figure 5.2*), the only form in which the core protein occurs outside the infected cell.

The precore product is translated from an initiation site a short distance upstream of that at the start of the core protein gene and is in the same reading frame. The extra sequence present at the N terminus of the precore protein directs this product into the endoplasmic reticulum in which it is truncated by proteolysis at both the N and C ends to give a 16 kD form which is then secreted into the blood. This form of the core protein does not have the self assembling, particle forming properties of the core protein proper and is found in large amounts in the

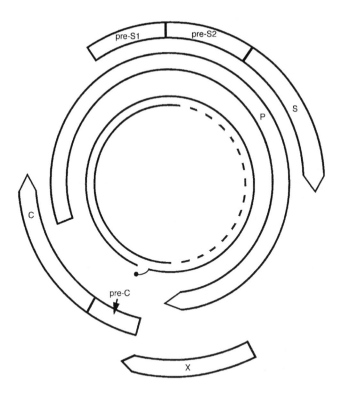

Figure 5.1:   Structure of the hepatitis B virus genome. The circular, incomplete double-stranded DNA as found in virus particles is represented by the single and dotted lines. It is converted into a complete closed circular structure upon infection of a new cell. The broad arrows represent the open reading frames coding for: Pre 1, Pre S2 and S, the various forms of the surface antigen protein; C the core and preC, the precursor to e antigen; P the viral polymerase enzyme; and X, the X protein.

blood of HBV infected patients. Despite its sequence identity to the core protein, the secreted version is antigenically distinct and is known as e antigen (eAg). The function of eAg in the biology of the virus is unclear but is probably related in some way to the avoidance of immune clearance of the virus during persistent infection. It has been suggested that eAg may play a role in the vertical transmission of infection by partially tolerizing the fetus *in utero* to infection. A further implication for a possible role of eAg in the immune evasion mechanisms used by the virus is suggested by the observation that mutant viruses which are unable to produce eAg often arise in patients who are beginning to develop an effective immune response.

The other structural proteins of the virus are three membrane glycoproteins, s (small), m (medium) and l (large), which are also a nested set sharing a common C terminal region. The m protein consists of HBsAg with an N terminal extension, the preS-2 region, while l is extended by preS-1 and preS-2. Complete virus

Table 5.2: HBV gene products and functions

Protein	Size (amino acids)	Properties and functions
e antigen	150	Secreted, truncated form of c antigen Role in immune evasion?
c antigen	183	Core protein Forms nucleocapsid
s antigen	226	Membrane protein, 50% of molecules glycosylated Major component of viral envelope Large amounts secreted as nonviral particles Role in immune evasion?
m	281	Membrane protein, 50% of molecules glycosylated s antigen with pre S2 N terminal extension Minor component of viral envelope Role in attachment and uncoating?
l	389-400	Membrane protein, 50% of molecules glycosylated s antigen with pre S1 + pre S2 N terminal extension Role in attachment and uncoating?
pol	845	Three domains — primer for DNA synthesis, polymerase, RNase H Copies pre-genomic RNA into genomic DNA
X	154	Affects transcriptional transactivation

particles, known as Dane particles, contain all three proteins in their outer envelope. In addition, large amounts of the s and m proteins are secreted into the blood in the form of empty membranous particles and tubules (*Figure 5.2*). Again the biological relevance of this phenomenon is unclear, but is probably involved in the maintenance of viral persistence. Since the outer surface of the Dane particle is composed of the s, m and l proteins, the receptor binding function of the virus must involve one or more of them. The unique portions of both the l and m proteins have been suggested to contain the receptor binding determinants of the virus, but there appears to be little consensus on both the definition of the receptor binding site on the virus or the cell receptor used by the virus. Interestingly, difficulties in identifying virus receptors have been encountered with all of the hepatotrophic viruses.

The largest ORF encodes the viral polymerase and occupies 80% of the virus genome. This protein has three distinct functional domains; an N-terminal primer protein which is covalently attached to the 5′ end of the negative strand DNA during viral replication, a central domain which has sequence motifs typical of nucleic acid polymerases, and a C terminal domain which has an RNase H function.

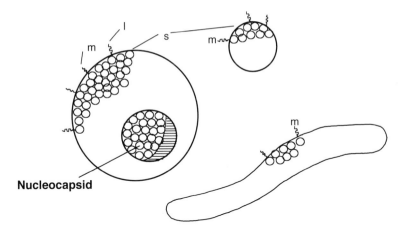

Figure 5.2: Hepatitis B virus related particles found in infected serum. Large quantities of S and M proteins are found as 23 nm spherical particles and tubules. The infectious Dane particles (42 nm) comprise the DNA containing nucleocapsid within a lipid envelope containing L, M and S proteins.

The shortest functional ORF encodes the X protein, which has been shown to effect transactivation although it is not itself a transcription factor. Instead, it appears to function by modifying the transcription initiating function of host factors. The role of the X protein in the viral replication is unclear, since its absence does not seem to influence the replication of the virus following transfection of viral DNA into cells *in vitro* yet it is essential for growth of the virus *in vivo*.

5.3.2 Hepatitis B virus: disease

The acute disease seen in HBV infected individuals ranges from clinically inapparant infection to fatal fulminant hepatitis. Similarly, chronic infections can vary greatly in their presentation from benign conditions through to chronic active hepatitis with sequalae of cirrhosis and liver cancer. In fact, of the estimated 350 million chronic carriers of HBV, 65 million are expected to die of chronic liver disease and it has been estimated by the WHO to be the ninth most important cause of death globally.

Although integration of the viral genome into the host cell DNA is not required for viral replication, as it is in the retroviruses, fragments of HBV DNA are commonly found to have been incorporated into host DNA in chronically infected patients. This occurs by a random, nonspecific mechanism and may play an important role in the development of hepatocellular carcinoma, which is frequently seen in long-term chronic carriers.

5.3.3 Hepatitis B virus: screening for antiviral compounds

The lack of cell culture systems which will support the full replication cycle of the virus is a complicating factor in the search for antiviral compounds. Although it is possible to replicate the virus in cells of hepatocyte origin following transfection with closed circular HBV DNA genomes, there are few reports of successful growth following infection with complete virus for reasons which are not understood. This restriction has been partially bypassed by the use of engineered cell lines in which tandem copies of the virus genome are integrated into the chromosomal DNA (*Figure 5.3*). In the normal replication of the virus a RNA 'pregenomic' intermediate is transcribed from the circular DNA template. During the transcription of this pregenomic RNA the polymerase ignores a termination signal present a short distance from the transcription initiation site on the first pass but recognizes it the next time round. The resulting RNA molecule thus has repeated sequences at its termini and these are important for the recircularization process involved in converting the RNA back into viral DNA. Consequently, it is necessary for the transformed cells to have tandem copies of the viral genome integrated into their chromosomal DNA so that the process of production of a pregenomic RNA can be mimicked on a linear template. Cell lines engineered in this way continuously produce low levels of virus and can thus be used as surrogates for a true infection system.

The rate of virus growth in these systems can be monitored by assessing the intracellular levels of HBV DNA genome replication intermediates by, for example, gel electrophoresis with detection by hybridization techniques. Alternatively, the virus particles secreted into the culture medium can be assayed by, for example, PCR methods. Although useful information can be obtained from these transformed cell systems, they are cumbersome, difficult to adapt for high throughput screening, and only partially representative of the virus growth cycle.

A cell free assay for the processive function of the viral polymerase is available using serum from chronic HBV carriers. If the virus in such samples is stripped of its envelope with mild detergents, the resulting core particles can proceed with the synthesis of the incomplete positive DNA strand if supplied with deoxynucleotide triphosphates and appropriate buffer conditions. The synthesis can be monitored by including a radioactively labeled precursor. Attempts to express an active form of the polymerase protein have met with minimal success and the reverse transcription process only seems to function properly within the context of the core particle.

The cell free assay using virus particle-derived cores can only be used to detect inhibitors of the viral polymerase and requires that nucleotide analogues to be tested must be converted to the triphosphate form. The transformed cell assay similarly reports on the viral polymerase function when intracellular viral DNA forms are used as the readout, but has the advantage that nucleotide analogs can be phosphorylated by the cell machinery. Assaying for extracellular secreted virus has the potential for identifying inhibitors of virus assembly as well DNA synthesis.

The transactivation activity associated with the X protein is another biochemical function for which assay development is possible. However, with the lack of a

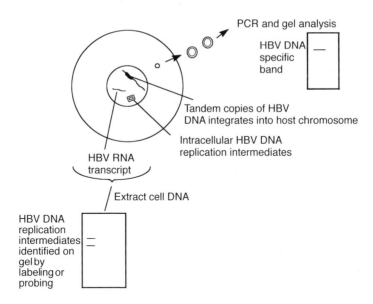

Figure 5.3: The use of a hepatocyte cell line stably transfected with tandem copies of the hepatits B virus DNA for the assay of antiviral compounds. Viral replication is initiated from the viral sequences inserted in the cell chromosomal DNA. This can be monitored by gel electrophoresis of intracellular replication intermediates or of PCR amplified portions of the virus genome present in released particles.

clear understanding of the precise role of the protein in the biology of the virus it is difficult to predict the likely effects that inhibitors of its function might have on chronic hepatitis.

5.3.4 Hepatitis B virus: testing candidate drugs

The only nonhuman species known to be susceptible to infection with HBV is the chimpanzee and so there is no convenient small animal model for the virus. There are, however, a number of related viruses affecting birds and small mammals, of which the mammalian examples are closest to human HBV. The most widely used of these is the Woodchuck virus, WHBV. This virus frequently causes chronic infection in the animals which invariably leads to hepatocellular carcinoma frequently linked with perturbations of proto-oncogenes, such as *c-myc* due to insertional mutagenesis. Similar alterations can occasionally be identified in human hepatocellular carcinomas.

Woodchucks are poor laboratory animals, particularly because of their require-ment for a hibernation period. However, a number of compounds have been tested in this model system; efficacy being measured as the reduction of viral load in the blood of chronically infected animals.

5.3.5 Hepatitis B virus: active compounds

Apart from natural immune modifiers, such as interferon (see below), most of the compounds which have been shown to have an antiviral effect on HBV are nucleoside analogs and, given that the DNA polymerase of HBV is a reverse transcriptase, as in the retroviruses, it is perhaps not surprising that there is a certain amount of overlap between compounds which are active against HBV and HIV. Unfortunately, many compounds which have been shown to have an inhibitory effect in *in vitro* assays have proved to be ineffective or to have unacceptable toxicity profiles *in vivo*. The dideoxynucleotide ddI, for example, is a chain terminator of DNA synthesis which has been shown to effective in inhibiting HBV replication in the transformed cell line assay but has not proved to be efficacious *in vivo*.

Problems associated with the toxicity of potential therapeutic compounds for viral hepatitis may well be exacerbated by the nature of the disease. The liver is the main site for the elimination of toxic materials from the body and it is therefore perhaps to be expected that detrimental side-effects are likely to be more apparent in patients with severe hepatitis. A tragic example is provided by the results of recent trials of the drug fialuridine (FIAU) (*Figure 5.4*). This compound was found to have antiviral activity against a number of herpesviruses and also against HBV, both in the *in vitro* transfected cell line assay and in the Woodchuck animal model. Initial trial studies in humans showed very good efficacy in terms of reducing the plasma levels of HBV as measured by viral DNA concentrations or by viral polymerase activity. In common with other trials with small molecule

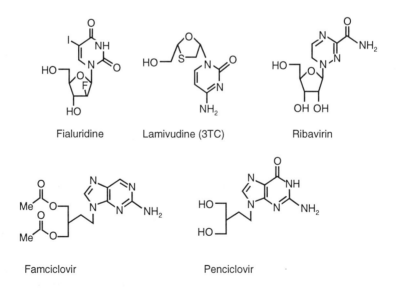

Fialuridine   Lamivudine (3TC)   Ribavirin

Famciclovir   Penciclovir

Figure 5.4: Some nucleoside analogs with antiviral activity.

inhibitors of HBV, the antiviral effects were not sustained on cessation of treatment. Further trials in which the duration of drug treatment was extended had to be curtailed when serious toxic side-effects became apparent. These included myopathy, lactic acidosis, peripheral neuropathy, pancreatitis and liver failure and the severity of the toxic effects were such that a number of patients died. The primary cause of this delayed toxicity was found to be mitochondrial damage associated with the incorporation of the drug into mitochondrial DNA, with consequent damage to the expression of mitochondrial genes. This effect had not been recognized in the *in vitro* toxicity assays that had been applied to the compound, but the incident served to highlight the necessity for thoroughly assessing future potential anti-HBV compounds for side-effects of this sort.

More encouraging results have been obtained in trials of another nucleoside analog in which the carbon atom at position 3 in the heterocyclic ring of the sugar moiety is replaced with sulfur. Lamivudine is the (−) enantiomer of 2′-deoxy-3′-thiacytidine (*Figure 5.4*) which has proved to be extremely effective in reducing the levels of markers of HBV (viral DNA and polymerase) in the blood of chronic carriers of the virus, as was seen with FIAU. However, in contrast to FIAU, lamivudine has proved to be extremely well tolerated over long periods of treatment, even in patients with active hepatitis. The drug has proved to be particularly useful in the control or prevention of reinfection of transplanted livers in HBV infected patients with disappearance of viral infection markers having been seen in a number of cases.

Famciclovir (*Figure 5.4*) is another nucleoside analog which appears in clinical trials to have interesting potential as an effective drug for the treatment of chronic HBV infection. This is the prodrug for the active compound, penciclovir (*Figure 5.4*), which was originally identified as a potential alternative to aciclovir for the treatment of herpesvirus infections. However, in contrast to aciclovir, penciclovir has also been shown to have potent antiviral activity against HBV both in the duck HBV model system and in human trials. Whereas aciclovir is not a substrate for cellular kinases, and so requires the thymidine kinase of herpesviruses to phosphorylate it to the active triphosphate form, penciclovir can be phosphorylated by cellular enzymes. It is this property of the compound that underlies its effectiveness against HBV since the virus does not encode a kinase activity. The specificity of the antiviral effect relies on differences in susceptibility of viral and host DNA polymerases to the phosphorylated form of the compound.

Despite the profound antiviral effects and acceptably low toxicity of some of these newer nucleoside analog drugs, their use does not generally result in clearance of infection and restoration of the chronic infection status resumes on cessation of drug administration. The effects of more protracted treatment periods on establishing curative responses are currently being evaluated and some patients have received continuous drug treatments in excess of a year without overt toxic consequences. However, as was to have been expected, drug resistant mutant viruses have begun to emerge in patients receiving prolonged treatments.

Lamivudine is effective against HIV as well as HBV but trials in AIDS patients have resulted in the rapid selection of drug resistant mutants. The mutations responsible for the resistant phenotype have been shown to effect an otherwise conserved amino acid motif — YMDD— which is thought to be a functionally important component of the active site of the reverse transcriptase enzyme of the virus. The mutations observed involve substitution of the tyrosine residue for isoleucine or valine. Interestingly, the same amino acid changes have been reported to occur in HBV variants resistant to lamivudine. Resistant viruses have also arisen in patients treated with famciclovir, but in this case the mutations responsible were in other regions of the viral polymerase than the YMDD motive. In view of these differences it will clearly be of great interest to investigate the potential synergistic effects of treating HBV infections with combinations of drugs with different precise sites of action, as is currently being studied in AIDS patients.

5.3.6 Hepatitis B virus: interferon

Interferon is a natural product that was first discovered by its antiviral effect as long ago as 1957. It is now known that there three major interferons, α, β and γ and that these are but three representatives of a large range of immunomodulatory molecules, the cytokines. IFN-α is the most widely used treatment for chronic HBV infection at present. The overall success rate, as assessed by clearance of viral infection, is approximately one-third of patients but this may be influenced in a minor way by alteration of the details of administration such as amount, frequency of dosing and duration of treatment It is therefore, not a perfect treatment but it is the best available at present and, moreover, analysis of the nature of the response in different patient groups provides some interesting indications of the nature of the virus/host relationship and the factors favorable to a sustained antiviral response. These in turn may be pointers to improved therapeutic approaches in the future.

IFN-α for clinical use is derived either from bacteria expressing recombinant human protein or from human lymphoblastoid cells which are induced to secrete interferon following infection with Sendai virus. Fifteen to twenty different species of IFN- α molecules are encoded in the human genome and the lymphoblastoid product is consequently a complex mixture of molecules. The recombinant products, however, contain a single IFN-α molecule. It is unclear why so many different interferon species are encoded and expressed, and if there is an advantage to be had from treating HBV with the natural mixture compared to a single molecule it is not overwhelming. One recognized advantage of the lymphoblastoid interferon is that it appears to be less immunogenic than the recombinant material in a minority of patients. A potential advantage of using the recombinant approach is that the molecule can be engineered in attempts to improve its efficacy but it is unclear at present whether this will work.

The antiviral effects of interferons are complex and operate at a number of levels. They can induce a variety of antiviral responses within the infected cell and can also influence immune recognition and so aid clearance of infection (*Table 5.3*). The effective components of the repertoire of interferon-induced responses which are responsible for the antiviral effect differs between viruses and

Table 5.3: Interferon induced effects

Synthesis of:	Activation of:	Inactivation of:	Effects on:
RNase L	RNase L by 2´-5´oligo A	Cellular and viral mRNAs	Viral and cell gene expression
2´-5´ oligo A synthetase	2´-5´ oligo A by dsRNA		
Protein kinase 67kD	Protein kinase 67 kD by dsRNA	Eukaryotic initiation factor 2 (eIF2)	Viral and cell gene expression
	Transcription of specific cellular genes		Induction of antiviral state
	MHC I presentation at cell surface		Immune enhancement
	MHC II presentation at cell surface		Immune enhancement

the specific mechanisms responsible for its anti-HBV activity are not fully understood. However, the features of patients who respond to interferon treatment with a sustained clearance of the infection are a low viral load in the blood and relatively high levels of liver enzymes, such as amino alanyl transferase. The latter feature is indicative of immune-mediated hepatocyte damage and implies, therefore, that there is a meaningful, if small, ongoing immune response. One effect of interferon treatment is to up-regulate the expression of major histocompatibility complex (MHC) proteins on infected hepatocytes, so increasing their recognition by T cells, and this is likely to be important in the mechanism(s) of the anti-HBV effect.

Interferons are induced naturally during viral infections and many of the 'flu-like' symptoms associated with the illness are, in fact, side-effects of interferon. Consequently, prolonged courses of interferon are often extremely unpleasant for patients and can lead to discontinuation of treatment.

5.3.7 Hepatitis B virus: immune globulins

Human immune globulin preparations have a specialized use in the management of HBV positive liver transplant patients to reduce the risk of infection of the donated liver. The cost of this treatment is high, up to that for the remainder of the transplantation process, and there is a great need for more cost effective alternatives. Some of the nucleoside analog drugs discussed above appear useful in this context and will probably replace the use of immune globulin in the future. Monoclonal antibodies directed against neutralization epitopes on the surface protein are potential alternatives to the use of human polyclonal immune globulin preparations and have been used in a limited number of trials.

5.3.8 Hepatitis B virus: conclusions

Effective treatment of chronic HBV infection remains a major challenge. Treatment with IFN-α is the oldest and most widely used therapeutic intervention but this is only effective in approximately one-third of patients. Moreover, it is associated with unpleasant side-effects and is expensive to produce and administer. Analysis of the profiles of successful responders to interferon treatment suggest that some, albeit low, immune response is an essential prerequisite for the successful clearance of infection by interferon. Consequently, therapeutic approaches which include an immunotherapeutic aspect are likely to be an important feature of future curative treatments. Advances in vaccine technology hold out the promise of improving on the inadequate immune response which allows the virus to establish persistent infection.

Despite early setbacks due to lack of *in vivo* efficacy or unacceptable or even fatal toxicity, there are now a number of small molecules which are looking promising as useful drugs. Predictably, drug-resistant viruses have begun to emerge, but it is too early to properly assess the potential impact of such mutants. However, their existence should encourage the investigation of combination treatments involving the simultaneous administration of compounds which act at different sites in the viral replication machinery, as is being pursued with the treatment of HIV infection.

5.4 Chronic viral hepatitis: hepatitis C virus

5.4.1 Hepatitis C virus: structure and replication

Following the development and application of diagnostic tests for hepatitis A and B viruses it became apparent that a proportion of transfusion-associated hepatitis was caused by further, as yet unidentified, agents. However, no virus could be grown from samples, which had been proven to have transmitted infection via blood donation, in a wide range of tissue culture systems. Chimpanzees were the only nonhuman species shown to be susceptible to the agent. These biological restrictions necessarily limited progress but, after many years of failure, the principal causative agent of nonA nonB transfusion-associated hepatitis (NANB TAH) was identified in 1989 by sophisticated cDNA cloning and expression techniques and termed hepatitis C virus (HCV).

HCV has a RNA genome approximately 9.3 Kb in length and sequence analysis showed that the genome organization was similar to that of viruses belonging to the family Flaviviridae, although the sequence homology with known members of the family was exceedingly low. The genomic RNA is of positive polarity and so can act directly as a messenger RNA for the production of viral proteins.

Because of this property infection can be initiated from the naked RNA genomes of positive strand viruses and it has recently been demonstrated that the RNA derived from molecular clones of HCV can, indeed, initiate infection when injected directly into the livers of chimpanzees. This observation will be of great importance to further studies on HCV.

The virus genome has a single ORF and the RNA is translated into a polyprotein of approximately 3000 amino acids. The polyprotein is processed into the mature functional viral proteins (*Table 5.4*) by a combination of host and viral proteolytic enzymes, as shown in *Figure 5.5*. The structural proteins of the virus are located within the N terminal third of the polyprotein and are cleaved by host signalase proteases. They consist of a core protein, which is presumed to assemble with the viral RNA into nucleocapsids, and two envelope glycoproteins, E1 and E2 The remainder of the polyprotein comprises the proteins involved in viral replication, which are processed by viral protease functions contained within the sequence. These nonstructural proteins are termed NS2–NS5, following the nomenclature used for the flaviviruses. In contrast to the flaviviruses, HCV appears to have no equivalent of the glycosylated NS1 protein.

Although there is still a great deal to learn about the mechanisms involved in the replication of HCV, a combination of comparative virology and molecular biology techniques has yielded much information on the functions of the nonstructural proteins of the virus. Because of the inability to grow the virus effectively in tissue culture the functions of the viral proteins have to be studied following their expression using recombinant DNA technology.

The obvious similarities in the overall organisation of the HCV genome to those of the flaviviruses, together with the occurrence of sequence motifs, allowed informed predictions of the specific functions of some of the HCV proteins to be made. The known activities of the viral proteins are given in *Table 5.4*. The predicted, and subsequently formally proven properties of some of the virus specified proteins immediately suggested potential targets for the development of antiviral compounds.

Table 5.4: HCV gene products and functions

Protein	Size (amino acids)	Properties and functions
Core	191	Nucleocapsid
E1	198	Envelope glycoprotein
		Forms heterodimer with E2
E2	340	Envelope glycoprotein
		Forms heterodimer with E1
NS2	297	Unknown
NS3	631	Serine protease
		NTPase/helicase
NS4A	52	Co factor for NS3 protease
NS4B	261	Unknown
NS5A	447	Unknown
NS5B	590	RNA dependent RNA polymerase

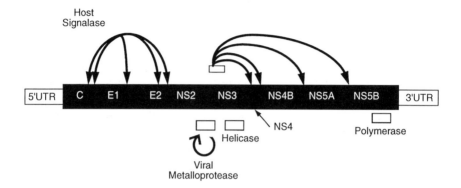

Figure 5.5: Diagrammatic representation of the genome of hepatitis C virus. The virus RNA is approximately 9.5 Kb in length with a long untranslated region (UTR) at each end. The protein product of the single long open reading frame is processed by host and viral enzymes into the mature structural (C, E1 and E2) and nonstructural proteins. The open boxes indicate the approximate positions of function related sequence motifs.

The serine protease function found to be associated with the N terminal portion of the NS3 protein was the first activity to be extesively studied. This enzyme is crucial for the virus as it is responsible for most of the cleavage events involved in the processing of the nonstructural portion of the viral polyprotein to release the functional mature products. There is also precedence in the HIV field for the successful development of antiviral compounds targeted against a viral protease. The specificity of substrate recognition by the NS3 protease is modulated by association with another viral protein, NS4A, and some cleavage sites are only cleaved by the complexed protease. Inhibition of this association would also be a possible stratagy for antiviral development.

The NS3 protein also has a helicase activity associated with the C terminal part of the protein and this is presumably involved in the process of viral RNA replication. The NS5B protein has a GDD motif typical of RNA polymerases and has, indeed, been shown to function as such in *in vitro* assays. Inhibitors against both the NS3 helicase and NS5B polymerase activities would be expected to interfere with viral replication and so be potential antiviral agents.

In addition to the protein coding region of the viral RNA, there are long untranslated regions (UTRs) at both the 5′ and 3′ ends of the molecule. The 5′ UTR is approximately 340 nucleotides in length and is one of the most highly conserved portions of the viral genome. It is considerably longer than the 5′ UTR of typical flaviviruses, which are approximately 120 nucleotides in length, and contains a number of AUG codons upstream of the AUG which initiates the translation of the long ORF. It also has a high degree of secondary structure which is even more highly conserved than the nucleotide sequence as most substitutions within base paired regions are matched by compensatory mutations which preserve base pairing. These features, which are also seen in the pestiviruses, are reminiscent of the 5′ UTRs of viruses of the picornavirus family, which have been shown to initiate protein translation by an unusual mechanism. This involves the direct association of ribosomes within the 5′ UTR, at a region termed the internal ribosome entry site (IRES), and bypasses the requirement for a capped free 5′ end to the messenger RNA. IRES elements are thus able to promote the initiation of translation of a downstream gene when they are inserted between cistrons in synthetic bicistronic messenger RNA (*Figure 5.6*). This functional assay has been applied to the 5′ UTR of HCV to formally demonstrate that it indeed can function as an IRES element.

The sequence at the 3′ end of the viral RNA also contains some interesting features, although even less is known about its role in viral replication. For a number of years it was thought that the 3 UTR consisted of a relatively short heteropolymeric stretch of sequence followed by a variable homopolymeric stretch of about 15 U residues. However, more stringent techniques have recently been used to show that the polymeric U sequence (admixed with a few C residues) is approximately 100 nucleotides long and that this is followed by a highly structured and highly conserved region of approximately another 100 residues. Such a highly structured region at the 3′ terminus of the RNA appears to be a general feature of flaviviruses and is most likely involved in the initiation of RNA replication.

5.4.2 Hepatitis C virus: disease

The true incidence of HCV infection only became apparent once the virus had been identified by molecular techniques and diagnostic reagents developed. It soon became apparent that the virus was responsible for approximately 90% of

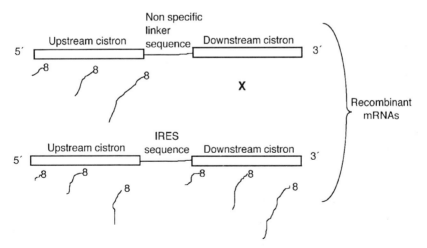

Figure 5.6: Recombinant bicistronic mRNAs. The upper molecule is translated to produce only the upstream cistron protein as the nonspecific sequence linking the two protein coding regions does not permit ribosomes to initiate translation of the downstream cistron. In the lower structure the presence of a specific viral sequence (IRES or Internal Ribosome Entry Site) between the cistrons allows both to be translated independently.

chronic NANB viral hepatitis. Furthermore, epidemiological studies show that there is 0.1–1% seropositivity in most parts of the world, although there is evidence for much higher levels of infection in some countries, and the majority of seropositive individuals are also positive for viral RNA. The virus is transmitted parenterally by blood transfusion, drug abuse, etc., but up to half of seropositive individuals have no known risk factors and how the infection is acquired in these people is unclear.

Clinically, the immediate consequences of infection with HCV are usually mild, in fact 70–80% of cases are asymptomatic. However, the majority of primary infections become established as long-term, usually life-long, chronic persistent infections and it is this propensity of the virus that underlies the development of serious liver disease long after the initial infection. It is the apparent ease with which the virus can initiate a persistent infection status that is perhaps its most intriguing feature. The mechanisms which allow the virus to escape immune elimination are not at all understood. It does not appear to be due to the paucity of an immune response, as seems to be the case with HBV, since both humoral and cell-mediated responses can be detected in persistently infected individuals and there is good circumstantial evidence that immune pressure drives antigenic evolution of the virus during chronic infection.

Despite the lack of symptomatic disease for long periods in most infected individuals, biopsy samples usually show some histological damage in the liver but it is still unclear whether the virus is directly cytopathic, or whether hepatocyte damage is immune-mediated, or whether a combination of these factors is involved. Whatever the mechanisms, it is probably the long-term damage to hepatocytes that ultimately leads to chronic active hepatitis, cirrhosis and hepatocellular carcinoma. Although there is a clear association of these serious liver diseases with infection with HCV, the prognosis for infected individuals is still unclear, principally because the long time interval between initial infection and the development of serious disease complicates epidemiological studies. Despite these difficulties in assessing the significance of HCV infection in individual patients, it is now the biggest single cause for liver transplantation.

5.4.3 Hepatitis C virus: screening for antiviral compounds

As with HBV, the intractable biological problems associated with attempts to culture the virus are a major complicating factor in the search for effective antiviral drugs against HCV. Although there are a few reports of reliable evidence for the *in vitro* propagation of the virus, the extent of replication is so low that PCR-based technology is required to demonstrate it and it is impracticable as the basis for a high throughput drug screening assay. Because of these restrictions, emphasis has been placed on the development of assays which are based on specific biochemical functions of virus proteins produced by recombinant DNA technology. Although the small size of the genome and our limited understanding of the detailed mechanisms of viral replication restrict the number of potential targets, there are at least five candidates.

The serine protease function associated with NS3 has received most attention as the basis for the development of antiviral drug screening assays. It was demonstrated early in the history of molecular biological studies of HCV that expressed portions of the polyprotein containing the sequence for NS3 were able to undergo proteolysis and that this activity was abolished if the predicted active site serine residue was mutated to an alanine. Furthermore, the addition of wild-type NS3 to polyprotein containing the mutated serine residue allowed the cleavages to occur, thus demonstrating that the enzyme could function in trans. From these basic observations assays were developed which followed the hydrolysis of an expressed portion of the polyprotein containing the cleavage site between NS5A and NS5B, which is the most easily cleaved *in vitro*, by the addition of purified NS3 in the presence of potential inhibitors. Further refinements of the assay (*Figure 5.7*) include the substitution of synthetic peptide substrates for expressed polyprotein, the dispensing of the C terminal portion of NS3, which does not contribute to the protease function and the inclusion of the part of NS4A which interacts with NS3 to modulate its activity. Although *in vitro* enzyme based assays like this can be useful in identifying inhibitory compounds, they fall far short of a full drug screening assay since factors such as cytotoxicity and accessibility of compounds to cells are not addressed and require further assays. Consequently, a number of potential cell-based assays designed to report cleavage due to NS3 protease in a readily measurable way are under development. Recently the structures of the NS3 protease alone or in combination with NS4 have been solved at high resolution by X-ray crystallography. This should aid the rational design of inhibitory compounds and potential antiviral drugs as it has with the AIDS virus, HIV.

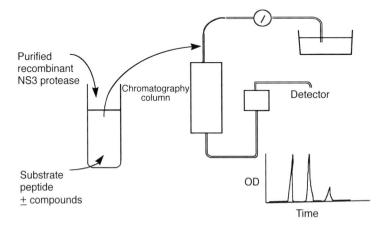

Figure 5.7: *In vitro* assay for viral protease function. Purified recombinant protease is mixed with peptide substrate with or without potentially inhibitory compounds. Samples are withdrawn at intervals and the conversion of peptide substrate into products is monitored by column chromatography.

The other known viral protease, which catalyzes the cleavage between NS2 and NS3, is another potential target since NS3-mediated proteolysis appears to be compromised if this cleavage does not occur. However, this function is much less well understood than that of NS3 and study of its potential as a therapeutic target is not as advanced.

Two known functions which are thought to be involved in replication of the viral genome are the helicase activity located in the C terminal portion of NS3 and the RNA polymerase activity associated with NS5B. *In vitro* assays for both of these activities are under development.

Finally, the IRES function associated with the 5′ UTR of the virus represents another potential target since this mechanism for the initiation of protein synthesis is not normally used by host cell messenger RNAs.

Another approach to the discovery of anti-HCV drugs is to use related viruses as surrogates in the anticipation that inhibitory compounds may also be active against HCV. The advantage of this approach is, of course, that viruses which can be easily propagated *in vitro* and which infect laboratory animal models can be chosen as surrogates. However, the problem remains of how to test potential drugs identified via this route against HCV. Also, the validity of any known viruses as surrogates for HCV is questionable given the slender homology it has with even the more closely related viruses such as the pestiviruses. A potential compromise is to construct artificial viruses in which replication is dependent on an introduced HCV-specific function, such as proteolysis. For example, it was recently reported that a recombinant poliovirus has been constructed in which the sequence coding for the NS3 protease of HCV is fused to the polyprotein coding region of poliovirus. This chimeric virus is only able to replicate if the added HCV component is cleaved autocatalytically from the polio virus polyprotein using the proteolytic activity of NS3. The ability of the virus to replicate and develop plaques is thus a marker of a functional protease and inhibitors of this function would render the virus inactive.

5.4.4 Hepatitis C virus: testing candidate drugs

As with HBV, there is no convenient animal model for the virus, the chimpanzee being the only known nonhuman host. Unlike HBV, however, there are no known animal viruses which resemble HCV. These problems, together with the difficulties associated with growing the virus *in vitro*, even in primary hepatocyte cultures, make the testing of candidate drugs against genuine HCV infection extremely difficult. Surrogate assays for specific HCV functions, as in the recombinant poliovirus model mentioned earlier, may be successfully developed but a test system which involves genuine HCV replication is preferable. Implants of infected human liver tissue into immunocompromised mice have been reported to continue virus production for some time but the difficulties involved in setting up such a model would probably severely restrict its use as a system for drug testing. In fact, direct testing in patients is the only effective route at present.

5.4.5 Hepatitis C virus: active compounds

The development of screening assays for potential antiviral compounds is an ongoing process and, as yet, there have been no reports of the identification of useful molecules. Ribavirin is a nucleoside analog (*Figure 5.4*) which has been shown have antiviral activity against a range of RNA viruses and has been used in clinical trials to treat chronic HCV infection with limited success. It appears to have no effect on the level of circulating virus, but there is often a reduction in the markers of active hepatitis. The use of ribavirin in conjunction with interferon in patients who did not respond to interferon has lead to the clearance of infection in some cases. The mode of action of ribavirin in this context is not known and it is possible, given the lack of effect on serum virus load when administered alone, that its effect is on the host rather than directly on the virus.

5.4.6 Hepatitis C virus: interferon

As with chronic HBV disease, the main therapeutic armament against HCV infection is IFN-α. However, the success rate of treatment is even less than that seen with chronic HBV infection. Approximately one-half of patients respond to interferon treatment with a reduction in virus levels and the serum enzyme markers of hepatitis. A large proportion of these patients revert to pre-treatment levels when interferon is withheld and the overall clearance rate is approximately 20%. Changing the dosing regime can marginally influence these figures but still the proportion of patients in whom a sustained response is achieved is disappointingly small.

It is not known which of the various antiviral effector mechanisms induced by interferon is responsible for its action against HCV. However, there is some correlation between the likelihood of a successful outcome of treatment and a low virus load in the blood. Virus of genotype 1b is often associated with higher viral loads than are seen with other genotypes and the prognosis for the efficacy of interferon treatment is generally poorer with these infections. Although there is much variation, the factors which are most indicative of a successful outcome of interferon treatment are low virus load and the absence of important liver pathology. This leads to the quandary that treatment is most likely to be successful in the least needy patients.

5.4.7 Hepatitis C virus: conclusions

There has been a very rapid advance in our knowledge and understanding of the virus since the first breakthrough of identifying and characterizing it was made in 1988. This knowledge is being applied vigorously to the development of assays for screening for molecules which can inhibit virus specific functions, and thus be candidate antiviral drugs, but the treatment procedures currently in use have been developed by empirical approaches. The success rate of these treatments is depressingly low, especially in those with the greatest clinical requirement for effective intervention and there is a great need for more effective treatment.

A small number of infections are successfully resolved and an understanding of the mechanisms underlying clearance of the virus in these cases could be crucial to the development of more effective therapeutic intervention. In addition, understanding of these cases could be important in the development of effective vaccines, which at present seem a remote possibility.

References

1. Hoofnagle, J.H. and Lau, D. (1997) *J. Viral Hepatitis* **4**, 41–50.
2. Clarke, B. (1997) *J. Gen. Virol.* **78**, 2397–2410.
3. Alter, H.J. (1995) *Blood* **85**, 1681–1695.

Chapter 6

Chemotherapy of human papillomavirus infections

6.1 Introduction

The papillomaviruses are a group of small nonenveloped double-stranded DNA viruses. They have been characterized from both humans and a growing range of other vertebrates including cattle, dogs, sheep, some avian species, mice and non-human primates. Some of the nonhuman papillomaviruses, in particular the bovine group (Bovine papillomavirus — BPV) have served as valuable study models and yielded much useful information on the molecular biology and pathobiology of these viruses.

Papillomaviruses are highly species specific. Currently there are no examples of a natural human papillomavirus (HPV) infection in another species and only one example in other animals — the nonproductive BPV infection of horses. They also have a highly restricted tissue tropism, exclusively infecting either squamous epithelial cells at either cutaneous or mucosal sites. Some HPVs are found at both cutaneous and mucosal sites [1].

The development of antiviral therapies against the human papillomaviruses requires appropriate *in vitro* and *in vivo* models and the restricted species and tissue specificity of these viruses has made this difficult. Study models are currently restricted to *in vitro* organotypic 'raft' cultures, and heterologous and homologous *in vivo* animal systems. Heterologous animal models include the severe-combined immunodeficient (SCID) and athymic mouse xenograft system, a mouse model grafted with syngeneic keratinocytes expressing human viral proteins, and more recently the transgenic mouse model where transgene expression is restricted to the epithelium by use of the human keratin 14 gene promoter. Homologous systems (surrogate models) employ animal papillomaviruses in their natural hosts and include bovine papillomavirus models, cottontail rabbit papillomavirus (CRPV) model, and canine oral papillomavirus (COPV) model [2]. A possible oral rabbit model has recently been described.

So far over 80 HPV genotypes have been isolated from humans and many of these have now been shown to be causative for specific pathologies. Infection may result in an inapparent and possibly latent infection, or alternatively it may result in either a benign lesion with varying morphology, or a proliferative lesion with varying risk of malignant progression. New HPV genotypes are identified on the basis that the nucleotide sequence within the complete L1 open reading frame (ORF) differs by more than 10%. HPV subtypes have also been identified. These have between 90 and 95% sequence similarity with the HPV prototype in the L1 ORF. A HPV variant is currently defined as having greater than 98% sequence identity with the prototype and significant differences in pathogenicity have recently been associated with these [3]. The basal cutaneous or mucosal epithelial cell is the initial target for the virus and while unproven, minor epithelial damage (exposure of the basal cell layer) is the most likely route of primary infection.

Cell surface receptor binding, epithelial cell entry, entry into the nucleus and uncoating are all undertaken by undefined mechanisms. The virus is able to bind to a wide range of cell types in addition to squamous epithelial cells and so the surface receptor is unlikely to be specific to the keratinocyte. Very recently, integrin α6 was identified as a candidate receptor. The virus is shed in squames. It is not cytolytic.

6.2 Genome organization and replication

The papillomavus genome length is approximately 8 Kb and contains three functionally distinct regions. These are the early region encoding genes involved in replication and transformation, the late region encoding two capsid proteins, and a regulatory region, (long control region — LCR), containing the viral origin of replication and transcriptional enhancer elements which are responsive to both viral and cellular factors. The LCR region also contains constitutive enhancer elements which have some tissue or cell type specificity and which are active in the absence of viral gene products. These enhancer elements are probably responsible for initial viral gene expression after virus infection and they are also largely responsible for the restricted tissue tropism seen with these viruses.

The early gene region comprises ORFs E1, E2 and E4–E7 and the late gene region comprises two ORFs which encode the major and minor capsid proteins (L1 and L2). L1 comprises approximately 80% of the total viral protein. The designation early or late gene reflects the position of the gene on the genome and need not reflect its time of expression during the viral life cycle.

All of the papillomaviral genes are encoded on one DNA strand and the position, the size, and function of the genes are well conserved amongst the various HPV types that have been studied thus far.

HPV gene expression is closely linked to the differentiation status of the infected epithelial cell. Different promoters and alternate RNA splice sites have been shown to be used depending upon the differentiation status of the infected cell. Early viral genes involved in viral gene regulation and DNA replication are expressed in the basal and spinous epithelial cell layer. Both early and late gene synthesis occurs in the more differentiated squamous cell layers and finally the capsid proteins are expressed and infectious virions assembled only in the most superficial fully differentiated squamous cell layers (*Figure 6.1*).

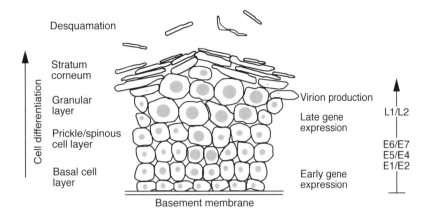

Figure 6.1: HPV gene expression in stratified epithelium.

The time course of viral DNA replication is similarly linked to the differentiation status of the cell. Following infection of the basal epithelial cell the viral genome may undergo a short amplification period, boosting the number of genome copies in the cell to 50–400. The genomes are then maintained episomally, replicating on average once per cell cycle. Evidence from recent studies with BPV indicates that the genome is stably maintained and partitioned between dividing cells. The switch to vegatative genome replication occurs as the infected cell differentiates and abundant copies of the viral genome are then produced for packaging into new virions. The switch from the maintenance to vegatative stages appears to be linked to terminal differentiation and growth arrest and the viral replication proteins (E1 and E2) are likely to be involved in this process. Several studies have indicated that replication proteins from one HPV genotype can initiate replication from the replication origin of another in various cell lines. In contrast to viral gene transcription which is highly tissue specific the replication machinery of the papillomaviruses therefore appears to be highly promiscuous [4].

HPV infection delays the normal differentialtion program of the cell. The result is a generalized hyperplasia typified by a number of histopathological changes. More specifically these include acanthosis (hyperplasia/thickening of prickle cell layer), parakeratosis (retension of nuclei in differentiated epithelial cell layers), pyknosis (nuclear thickening/increase in nuclear density), and koilocytosis (formation of large perinuclear cavities). While these histologic changes are characteristic of HPV infection viral particles and antigen are only detected in a small proportion of these cells. The molecular basis for these virus induced changes remains unclear.

6.3 Papillomavirus proteins

The E1 protein is an ATP-dependent DNA helicase and binds sequence specifically to the viral origin of DNA replication. It is the only papillomavirus protein that is directly involved in DNA replication. E1 also binds to a subunit of the host cellular DNA polymerase α – primase complex and it may therefore play a pivotal role in the assembly of the replication complex of proteins at the viral origin of replication.

The E2 protein is a sequence-specific DNA binding protein with important functions in both viral replication and transcription. Three species of E2, generated by use of alternate splice sites or promoters have been identified in the BPV system. E2 has been shown to repress expression of the HPV-16 E6 and E7 genes and deletion or disruption of E2 frequently occurs in transformed cell lines and invasive HPV disease.

The E4 gene is located in the early region of the genome and multiple E4 species are found in infected cells. However, it is expressed late and coincident with the the onset of productive (vegatative) viral replication. In some cases it has been associated with the collapse of the cellular cytokeratin network. Its precise role is unclear.

E5 has weak oncogenic potential. It appears to block the down-regulation of the epidermal growth factor (EGF) receptor by binding to vacuolar ATPase. This results in a reduction in the acidification of endosomes and this may then lead to increased amounts of epidermal growth factor receptor (EGFR) recycling back to the cell surface. EGF is a mitogen in keratinocytes and E5 may provide infected cells with a proliferative advantage. The E5 gene of HPV-16 has recently been shown to repress the expression of the tumor suppressor gene *p21*. The full range of its activities are unclear.

HPV E6 and E7 proteins are transforming proteins and have important roles in both replication and the development of cervical carcinoma [5]. They compromise the normal regulation of the host cell cycle by sequestering two key host proteins — pRB and p53. E6 binds to p53 and both blocks its transcriptional regulatory activity and targets it for rapid ubiquitin-mediated proteolysis. By binding to pRB the E7 protein blocks pRB-mediated negative regulation of the G1/S cell cycle check point. Taken together, blocking both pRB and p53 removes both a natural block in the cell cycle and the p53-mediated DNA damage repair pathway. Both proteins share the ability to allow cell cycle progression despite cellular DNA damage.

The binding affinities of the E6 and E7 proteins for p53 and pRB are not equal between the different HPV genotypes. A small subset of HPV genotypes are frequently associated with cervical cancer and the E6 and E7 proteins from these genotypes bind with high affinity to p53 and pRB. The E6 and E7 proteins from HPV genotypes that have infrequent association or no association with malignant disease either bind weakly or do not bind at all to p53 and pRB. These differences in relative binding affinities between the HPV genotypes determine their different transforming potential and the HPVs have correspondingly been designated high-, intermediate- and low risk genotypes. There is a similar correlation between p53 and pRB binding affinity and the ability of an HPV genotype to immortalize primary human fibroblasts.

HPV-mediated malignant transformation in cervical epithelia only occurs in a minority of infections and only the restricted 'high risk' subset of HPV genotypes are involved. In malignant lesions the HPV genome is often (but not always) shown to be integrated into host DNA. Integration has often been shown to disrupt the E1/E2 gene region with concomitant loss of E6 and E7 transcriptional control. E6 and E7 are then expressed at high levels and their continued expression is required for maintenance of the transformed phenotype. However, while E6 and E7 are necessary they are not sufficient for transformation. High grade cervical lesions and invasive cervical cancer are characterized by aneuploidy and chromosomal abberations and these changes are likely to contribute to the malignant process.

Transformed epithelial cells are nonproductive lesions and so the transformation process itself serves no useful purpose for the virus. The predominant role of E6 and E7 is to activate cellular genes involved in DNA replication and so generate a permissive environment in an otherwise quiescent cell. These proteins are not expressed in noncycling differentated epithelial cells where abundant viral DNA synthesis is known to occur. Host cellular replication proteins are essential components of HPV DNA replication.

6.4 Pathobiology

The human papillomaviruses can be divided into cutaneous genotypes which cause predominantly benign skin warts of varying morphology, and mucosal types associated with benign and premalignant lesions and cervical cancer.

6.4.1 Cutaneous genotypes

The cutaneous HPV group currently comprises more than 30 genotypes. These include HPVs 1, 2, 3 and 4 which are known to cause plantar warts mainly on soles of feet, common warts mainly on the hands, flat warts around the knees, arms and face, and mosaic warts on feet and hands. HPV-7 is particularly prevalent in warts found among meat handlers, fishmongers, poultry workers, and butchers (also known as Butcher's warts). This virus is virtually absent in warts isolated fom the general population.

Extensive cutaneous HPV lesions occur in epidermodysplasia verruciformis (EV), a rare life long skin disease with a high risk of malignant tranformation. Patients are unable to resolve the warts that develop and some of these may become malignant (squamous cell carcinoma — SCC). HPVs 5 and 8 are frequently associated with EV lesions that develop in this way and exposure to strong UV appears to be involved in the malignant transformation process. Interestingly while multiple HPV types are found in EV patients (at least 20) many of these occur only rarely in healthy individuals indicating an immunologic basis for the underlying disease [6].

Cutaneous warts are generally self-limiting proliferative lesions and about two-thirds will regress spontaneously after a period of several years. They are most prevalent in older school children and young adults. The incidence then declines and this may reflect acquired immunity and/or reduced exposure to the virus.

6.4.2 Mucosal genotypes

The mucosal group of papillomaviruses include more than 25 types which infect the genital tract (reviewed in [7]). Less common are other types which infect the oral cavity, respiratory tract and conjunctiva.

The clinical repercussions of HPV infection in the genital tract are variable. In both males and females infection may result in the formation of benign warts (genital warts — condyloma acuminata) which often resolve spontaneously. In females infection may be inapparent and without cytologic abnormality or it may be manifest as a mild disturbance of the cervical epithelia which if left untreated can develop into moderate and then sometimes severe cytologic abnormality. Eventually, albeit infrequently, invasive cervical cancer may develop and while disease occurs most frequently in the cervix (cervical neoplasia/cancer), lesions and subsequent cancer may also develop in the vagina, vulva, anus and penis.

To facilitate diagnosis the severity of the cytologic abnormality has been graded. Condylomata or mild cytologic abnormality are low grade cytologic disturbances of the lower third of the cervical squamous epithelia. These are described as low grade squamous intraepithelial lesions (SIL). High grade SIL includes lesions involving up to two-thirds or the whole of the epidermis and is used to define severe cytology and invasive disease/cancer. Preinvasive disease can also be classified as cervical intraepithelial neoplasia (CIN) — again with increasing severity grades; mild cytology (CIN1), moderate cytology (CIN2), severe cytology and invasive cancer (CIN3).

Epidemiologic studies have established a clear genotypic correlation with the severity of cytologic abnormality. Human papillomaviruses have correspondingly been graded as low, intermediate, and high risk HPV types. High risk types include HPV-16 and HPV-18, and these are frequently found in high grade precancerous disease and invasive cervical cancer (squamous cell carcinoma of the cervix). Low grade CIN containing high risk HPV types have a higher risk of developing into high grade disease and invasive cancer. HPV-16 is found most frequently (approximately 50% of cases) and HPV types 16, 18, 45 and 56 are together found in nearly 75%. HPV-18 appears to be associated with the more agressive and rapidly progressing tumors. The risk of progression from low grade CIN to to high grade CIN and invasive cancer correlates with viral load, duration of disease as well as HPV genotype.

HPV types 33 and 35 are also found in cervical cancers but much less frequently and so are regarded as of moderate or intermediate risk. Low risk types are rarely found in invasive cancers but when they are they are frequently shown to have acumulated mutations that may have contributed their malignant potential. Interestingly some HPV types that are frequently associated with condyloma have occasionally been found in CIN.

Genital HPV infections peak in early adulthood and appear to be equally prevalent in both men and women. Although the majority of cases of cervical neoplasia are the result of prior infection with HPV most initial infections do not lead to a diagnosed cytologic abnormality. When it does occur however, it is usually as a low-grade lesion (CIN1) and this becomes apparent 1–2 years after initial infection. Regression of CIN is common and can occur over the course of several months to 1 or 2 years. In one study 62% of CIN1 cases regressed, 22% persisted and 16% progressed to CIN3 over a period of 4 years. A high percentage of men whose female partners have CIN have been shown to have penile lesions (penile intraepithelial neoplasia — PIN), containing the same HPV type. HPV-16 is associated with a significant proportion of PIN.

CIN1 may deteriorate if left untreated and preinvasive disease (CIN3) can develop, typically within 5–7 years. Interestingly about 5% of infected women appear to develop CIN3 without apparent precient CIN1 or CIN2. While this might appear to be an atypical sequence of events it should be remembered that the cervical epithelium may have several distinct loci of infection and these neoplasia may progress at different rates. Multiple HPV infections of the cervix have been identified in ~25% of women.

HPV-related neoplasia at other sites in the genital tract, vulva, vagina and perineum are less frequent than those occuring in the cervix but HPV-16 is again predominant. HPV is also frequently associated with adenocarcinoma but unlike other HPV infected neoplasia where HPV-16 is most prevalent, in adenocarcinoma HPV-18 is the most common HPV type isolated.

The majority of genital warts (concylomata acuminata) contain HPV types 6 and 11 but types 42, 43, 44, 55, 57 are also associated. HPV-16 occurs in a small percentage of genital warts. Warts generally occur in several sites in infected individuals and more than 60% of patients with partners having condyloma develop genital warts with an average incubation period of 3 months.

There are two other rare variants of genital warts and these have significant malignant potential. Bowenoid papulosis is associated with mucosal types including HPV-16 and HPV-18 and giant condyloma (Buschke–Lowenstein) tumor, (associated with HPV types 6 and 11) ulcerates and infiltrates deeply. The rate of malignant progression in giant condyloma has been reported at 56%.

Papillomas occuring in the respiratory tract (laryngeal papillomatosis) are rare but they are debilitating and difficult to treat. Papillomas typically develop in the larynx. They can be removed surgically but recurrence is frequent and spread of the virus to other sites (trachea, lungs, nose) is common. HPV-6 and HPV-11 are almost exclusively associated with respiratory papillomas and in children maternal transmission (passage through an infected birth canal) is a likely cause. The condition can occur in adults and when it does the same genotypes predominate.

It is now accepted that nonsexual transmission of both high and low risk HPV types can occur. Mothers can transmit HPV to the infant even when her HPV infection is subclinical and the virus may persist for the first 2 or 3 years of life.

6.5 Prevalence of HPV disease

HPV prevalence in the genital tract of college women has been reported at 46% in the US, incidence peaking in 15–25 year olds who are sexually active. Infection is often transient lasting only a few months but persistent infections can occur in older women and in those infected with high risk HPV types. The prevalence of HPV in males is similar to that seen in females and there is clear evidence that in some countries the prevalence of HPV in both sexes is increasing.

Condylomata acuminata is a significant health problem with over one million new cases reported annually. It is the most common sexually transmitted viral disease in the UK and US and the incubation period can be long. Over 60% of the sexual partners of HPV infected individuals develop lesions within 4 weeks to 8 months.

World-wide cervical cancer is the most prevalent malignancy in women with over 440 000 new cases of cervical cancer occurring annually. In the developed countries it makes up over 7% of all female cancers with over 4500 deaths in the US each year. The prevalence of HPV detected in cervical carcinoma is more than 80% detected. The incidence of HPV in women in the US is increasing and one estimate of spending on detection and treatment in the US in 1994 was 6 billion dollars.

Significant mucosal and cutaneous HPV disease occurs in HIV patients with advanced disease and in immune suppressed patients such as solid organ transplant patients. HPV infection of the anus is common in homosexual men.

6.6 Diagnosis

Subclinical infections are currently defined as those that become visible after application of 5% acetic acid. White patches on the epithelium are then visible (acetowhitening), usually after examination under magnification with a colposcope. This type of subclinical lesion is much more prevalent than clinical (visible) disease. However, not all acetowhite lesions are HPV related. Other skin conditions and allergic reactions may also give an acetowhitening response.

Cytologic evidence of HPV infection forms the basis of ongoing mass screening program (Papanicolaou smear diagnosis). However, the correlation between cytology screening and detection of HPV DNA is less than 100% and false positive tests are not uncommon. An oligonucleotide hybrid-capture detection test has been developed and the the clinical use of DNA hybridization and PCR tests for the management of HPV disease are being evaluated. It is very unlikely that these tests alone will completely replace cytologic observation in the management of HPV disease. Currently, accurate diagnosis still requires a combination of histologic examination, clinical enquiry and virological testing.

6.7 Therapy

While there is currently no proven antiviral therapy there are a number of chemotherapeutic and surgical treatment options. Current treatments aim to eliminate the signs and symptoms of HPV disease and do not always eliminate the

HPV DNA itself. This often leads to recurrent disease and represents one of the major limitations of these methods. The success of surgical treatments, cryotherapy, laser vaporization, and surgical intervention, are dependent upon the resources and skill of the practitioner, as well as viral load, anatomical site, HPV genotype, age of wart/lesion, and immunologic status. Chemotherapeutic treatments suffer from a lack of specificity. In totality these factors result in highly variable success rates both in eliminating the disease symptoms and thereafter in reducing the frequency of recurrent disease.

Using PCR and hybridization procedures HPV DNA has been shown to be present in normal tissue adjacent to infected lesions and warts and failure to eliminate this virus will often result in recurrent disease. Most recurrent disease does develop in and around previously treated disease areas.

6.7.1 Current treatment options

Clinically the importance of treating external anogenital HPV infections are fourfold, relief of symptoms, the risk of transmission to sexual partners, the risk of developing malignancy and the risk of transmission to neonates. Since current evidence indicates that asymptomatic but HPV positive individuals do not transmit virus between sexual partners management of subclinical infection is not undertaken [8]. Therapy is therefore restricted to patients with clinical disease (visible lesions).

The treatment options for genital warts are not limited [9]. Liquid nitrogen, 50–80% bichloroacetic or trichloroacetic acid solution, anticancer agent 5-fluorouracil (5FU), the antimitotic podophylotoxin, and the interferons have all been used topically for the treatment of localized exophytic warts. These treatments are often only partially effective, and recurrence rates of greater than 50% after 1 year are frequently reported. High recurrence rates are caused by several factors — the inherent lack of efficacy with the treatment, repeat infection, the long incubation period of HPV, missed lesions, deep lesions, and the failure to clear HPV DNA from tissue surrounding the wart.

Exophytic lesions can resolve spontaneously without treatment and in 20–30% of patients this often occurs within a few months. However, this too can be problematic since a wart that does not resolve naturally can often lead to the development of more warts that are larger and heavily keratinized, making subsequent topical treatments correspondingly less effective. Early treatment of warts is therefore prudent and warts present for less than 1 year have been shown to respond to relatively few or even single treatments by a number of different treatment options.

Bichloroacetic acid and trichloroacetic acid solutions are dessicants and must be applied carefully to warts/lesions to avoid normal skin tissue. Burning will occur but this can be avoided by the use of topical anesthetics. None the less they are safe to use during pregnancy, and on warts within the vagina by careful application using colposcopy. Repeat treatments are usually required.

Cryotherapy with liquid nitrogen has been regarded as the safest and most effective treatment for genital warts. It has a reported success rate of > 70%, but multiple treatments are ususally necessary and most patients experience moderate pain during and after treatment. It is safe for use in the early stages of pregnancy and it is also used to treat CIN.

5-Fluorouracil inhibits nucleic acid synthesis and has been used for many years for the treatment of HPV disease. It is not FDA approved. Variable hypersensitivity reactions and ulceration may occur and it is teratogenic so many women are contra-indicated. Its success rate is reported at 40–68% with 0–10% recurrence after 6–12 months. Application is topical as a 5% 5FU cream.

Podophyllin has also been used topically. It is an antimitotic resin extract from the root of the May apple plant. Again, success rates vary greatly and both local and systemic side-effects following repeat use have limited its effectiveness. As with the dessicants clinical benefit is only evident several days after use and sloughing of the treated tissue will occur. Podophyllin contains variable amounts of the active ingredient podophylotoxin, so toxic side-effects are correspondingly variable. It cannot be used during pregnancy or intravaginally and side-effects (systemic neurologic and bone marrow toxicity) can occur if used repeatedly or excessively.

Podophylotoxin is the active ingredient of podophyllin. It has a low potential for systemic toxicity and higher success rate than podophyllin. Recurrence rates, however, are comparable to those with podophyllin. Recently available as a 0.5% cream (Condylox) it has a stable shelf-life and is recommended for home use. Repeat treatments are required daily with treatment free days between but heavily keratinized warts of long standing do not absorb well and correspondingly to not respond well. Complete clearance has been reported in about 50% of women who complete the recommended course of treatment. Recurrent leasions and primary treatment failures are often treated by destructive ablative or surgical methods and/or interferon therapy.

CO_2 laser therapy is used to treat both exophytic warts and CIN, and it has been recommended for the management of refractory or extensive HPV disease. The CO_2 laser destroys infected tisssue by vaporization and then delayed tissue necrosis. For a skilled practitioner who can control the the width and depth of tissue destruction there is virtually no scarring, healing is rapid, and the procedure can access otherwise inaccessible infected areas. In one recent study of 32 HPV-positive women treated all became HPV-negative and remained negative during the follow up period of 5 years. Interestingly, 100% spontaneous regression was seen in the control group (5 women) within 12 months. Another report showed that in 199 men with condylomatous lesions which had not responded to other treatments CO_2 laser therapy was completely successful in >80% of cases after just one treatment. Other reports are not so encouraging and have indicated complete clearance rates for exophytic warts at between 20 and 80%. Infectious virus has been detected in laser plume.

Other surgical methods, electroexcission, electrodessication, loop excission, and electrocautery can be similarly effective. Surgical methods are often used where other treatments have failed and cost/benefit to the patient is usually considered when referal for surgical methods are required.

6.7.2 Interferon therapy

Each of the three groups of interferons (α, β, γ), and both recombinant and natural interferons have been used to treat HPV disease. Both topical, intralesional (injection), and systemic routes of administration have been used (reviewed in [10]).

Efficacy is again highly variable. Complete clearance rates using natural and recombinant intralesional IFN-α in uncontroled trials have been reported at between 23 and 100%. One double blind study involving 86 patients did show a clear benefit with complete clearance rates in treated and placebo group after 3 months of 62 and 21% respectively. Other controled double-blind trials have shown no significant difference between IFN treated and control groups. Increased dose tends to improve clinical outcome. At high doses systemic monotherapy with IFN-α has proven 100% effective but adverse drug reactions required dose reductions during the studies.

IFN-β has recently been shown to be effective for treatment of CIN. Combined intralesional and systemic administration was more effective than either route alone. About 20% of patients did not respond and about 10% of patients had recurrence. This is in agreement with other reports and similar to efficacies reported with IFN-α treatment.

Data on IFN-γ monotherapy is limited but there is some evidence that it may be useful in the treatment of refractory genital warts.

Interferon treatment does appear to potentiate the effect of other treatments and combination therapy, for example IFN-α and laser therapy have been shown to be effective in reducing recurrence in patients with recalcitrant condylomata acuminata. The adverse effects of IFN treatment depend upon dose and route of administration. Intralesional application can be associated with pain at the site of inoculation unless volumes are small and doses greater than one million units (1 MU) frequently result in flu-like symptoms. Higher doses, greater than 5MU may result in nausea, vomiting, diarroea, peripheral neuropathy and certain patient groups, for example those who are pregnant, transplant patients and those with cardiovascular disease may be contraindicated. Topical application does not appear to have significant side-effects.

Overall the interferons do appear to show promise for the treatment of HPV disease. Between 40 and 60% of patients respond to injected IFNs and it is generally the higher doses that have proven most effective. Topical application is not as effective as systemic and combination therapy is clearly more effective than IFN montherapy. Optimal treatment parameters, route of admistration, dosing regimen and IFN formulation still need to be clearly defined and this will require further controlled testing. In general IFN treatment is less effective in immunocompromised HIV patients and in patients infected with the high risk genotypes HPV-16 and HPV-18.

6.7.3 Future treatments

New therapies (*Table 6.1*) for HPV disease will need to address the life cycle

Table 6.1: Products in development

Product name	Route of administration	Active component	Company/ Instituion	Status
Accusite	Injection	Fluorouracil/ epinephrine	Matrix Pharms, US	Launched UK
Imiquimod	Topical	Imidazaquinolone	3M Pharms, US	Launch 1997
Condolyx[a]	Topical	Podophylotoxin	Oclassen Pharms, US	Launched
Forvade	Topical	HPMPC	Gilead, US	Phase I/II
b		Ribozyme	Various	Preclinical
HYB 101400	Topical	Anti-sense oligonucleotide	Hoffman La Roche/ Hybridon Inc.	Preclinical
Intron A[a]	Injection	Recombinant interferon alpha-2b	Schering-Plough	Launched
Alferon N[a]	Injection	Human leukocyte-derived interferon	Interferon Sciences, US	Launched
b	Vaccine	Virus-like particle	Merck	Phase I Q2/97
MEDI-501	Vaccine	Virus-like particle	MedImmune	Phase I Q1/97
GENEVAX	Vaccine	Naked DNA	Apollon/Wyeth Ayerst	Preclinical
b	Vaccine	Naked DNA	Merck/Vical	Preclinical
TA-HPV	Vaccine	Vaccinia encoding HPV-16 E6 and E7	CANTAB Pharms, UK	Phase I/II
TA-GW	Vaccine	Fusion protein (L2/E7)	CANTAB Pharms, UK/SmithKline Beecham	Phase I/II
b	Vaccine	HPV-16 GST/E7 fusion protein	Brisbane, Australia	Phase I
b	Vaccine	HPV-16 E7 peptides	University Hospital Leiden	Phase I/II

[a] New combination treatments using these products both with and without surgical procedures are being explored.

[b] Product name/information unavailable.

with highly specific modalities if they are to improve upon current treatments. Despite the practical difficulties and limitations of current *in vitro* and *in vivo* models, enough information about critical viral functions is now available in order to concieve of rational ways of developing HPV specific antiviral agents against a subset of the HPV gene products [11]. Screening systems designed to discover small molecule inhibitors of the viral replication proteins E1 and E2 have recently been reported [12]. Of particular interest has been the helicase activity of the E1 protein but while an attractive target for antiviral chemotherapy, expressing enough soluble protein for *in vitro* drug screening has proven problematic. There is also some interest in specifically targetting the E6 mediated proteolysis of p53 via the ubiquitin pathway and the E7 protein interaction with the host cellular pRB protein is also a potential target. For both of these viral proteins their interface with the host protein may be an effective starting point for the discovery and development of inhibiting molecules. Targeting the biochemical activities of other papillomarvirus proteins must await a more complete understanding of their functions.

New drug discovery approaches include anti-sense and antigene technology. Theoretically these technologies could yield highly specific compounds by specifically targeting HPV RNA and DNA molecules. An anti-sense oligonucleotide (ISIS 2105) targeted to the HPV E2 mRNA of HPV-6 and HPV-11 has been shown to be efficacious *in vitro* but development was discontinued, reportedly because effective drug concentrations could not be maintained in the skin. Administration of the anti-sense oligonucleotide was by local injection after surgical removal of wart tissue. More recently a second anti-sense oligonucleotide (HYB 101400), targeted to the 5′ end of the E1 mRNA has shown promise by reducing viral load and wart size in a human foreskin renal xenograft nude mouse model. The 5′ end of E1 is highly conserved between the low risk genital HPV and preclinical testing is ongoing. Preclinical testing of a number of different ribozyme constructs is also underway. HPV antigene approaches which target DNA directly with triple-helix forming oligonuceotides whilst showing promise *in vitro* have been proven in principle only.

Other new developments include Accusite, an injectable gel for genital warts. The active ingredient is 5FU but it also contains a sustained release biodegradable gel with the vasoconstrictor epinephrine to maintain local concentrations of the drug. Phase II data indicated that four to five weekly treatments usually clears about 75% of injected genital wart lesions. About 60% of warts that clear completely remain clear during a 3 month follow-up. Accusite has recently been launched in the UK.

Cidofovir (HPMPC), a mononucleotide analog with demonstrated activity against several herpesviruses is also being developed as a topical gel formulation (Forvade) for genital warts. In a phase I/II trial 64% of enroled AIDS patients with genital warts showed a complete or partial clearance of the warts. A phase II trial in immunocompetent patients with genital warts is ongoing. Forvade is also being evaluated for efficacy against HPV-associated CIN.

Imiquimod is an inducer of IFN-α, TNF and other cytokines and it appears to induce local inflammatory responses. It has recently completed phase III trials as a 5% topical cream. Genital wart clearance rates of 56% for three times weekly and 71% for daily administration have been reported. Recurrence rates were 13% and 19% respectively. Complete clearance of warts can take several weeks.

6.8 Vaccines

One of the most promising and intensively studied areas relates to HPV vaccines. There is much commercial interest in this area and both therapeutic and prophylactic vaccine approaches are being developed [13].

A number of studies and observations have collectively indicated that a vigorous immune response may resolve existing HPV infection. Histologic observations of lymphotrophic infiltration at the base of resolving warts was an early indicator of the involvement of the cell-mediated immune response. Genetically and iatrogenically immunosuppressed individuals appear to be vulnerable to HPV disease, and leukemia and AIDS patients are also more susceptible. Surgical removal of warts often results in regression of warts at other sites and autogenous vaccination of humans using material derived from surgically excised warts has been reported to be highly effective in preventing recurrent lesions.

Much of the rationale for the current vaccine work is based upon animal model studies and a knowledge of both the site and function of HPV proteins in the infected epidermis. Since the E6 and E7 proteins are required to maintain the transformed phenotype therapeutic vaccines aimed at controling HPV-induced tumors have focused on both of these proteins. Correspondingly, E1 and E2 may be appropriate therapeutic targets in genital warts since these proteins are made in the infected dividing basal epithelial cell. The capsid proteins L1 and L2 are the targets of choice for a prophylactic vaccine and neutralizing antibody to capsid proteins should block viral infection. There is good animal model evidence to indicate that this does happen.

On a more cautionary note recent studies indicated important differences in the host immune response to genotypic viral variants compared to the prototype virus. For example, an amino acid substitution identified in the HPV-16 E6 protein may influence CTL recognition of invasive cervical carcinomas. This may provide a mechanism for escape from immune surveillance and this has important implications for vaccine development [20].

6.8.1 Therapeutic vaccines

To be successful a therapeutic vaccine must invoke an HPV-specific cytotoxic-T cell (CTL) response (MHC class I pathway), and/or a delayed-type hypersensitivity (DTH) response (MHC class II pathway). Consequently, the therapeutic vaccine approach has sought to identify and invoke these responses.

Early results have been encouraging. E6 and E7 proteins have been shown to be tumor rejection antigens in animal models (rats and mice). In the murine model E6 specific CD8+ CTL has been generated *in vitro* from spleen cells derived from the E6 immunized mice and an *in vitro* CD4-mediated CTL response has been demonstrated against E6 expressing syngeneic keratinocyte skin grafts in mice. In other animal model studies E1, E2 and E6 protein in CRPV, and BPV-2 L2 and BPV-4 E7 protein in cattle have all been shown to promote early regression of warts [14]. Interestingly, L2 may have utility as both a therapeutic and a prophylactic vaccine the former mediated perhaps by a bystander killing mechanism.

CTL epitopes on human papillomavirus E6 and E7 proteins have been investigated and mapped using a variety of *in vitro* methods and some of these have proven effective in mouse tumor models. CTL epitopes have also recently been mapped on HPV-16 E1 and E2 proteins. The immunogenicity of a HPV-16 E7 peptide has been shown to correlate with the affinity of the peptide for MHC class I molecules and both these and other studies have formed the basis for a peptide based phase I vaccine trial in end stage cervical cancer patients. Two E7 peptides with an unrelated peptide designed to ellicite a helper T-cell response have been injected with an oil-based adjuvant [15].

Other studies have been less encouraging, indicating that the level of E7 protein generated in an infected keratinocyte may determine either an inflammatory DTH response, or an unresponsive tolerance. Uncoupling the negative regulation of *E6* and *E7* gene expression by E2 and boosting their expression may therefore constitute a viable target for antiviral chemotherapy.

Nonpeptide based therapeutic vaccine trials are also ongoing. These include a vaccinia recombinant virus encoding HPV-16 and HPV-18 E6 and E7 proteins for cervival cancer and an HPV-11 E7/L2 bacterial fusion protein for genital warts. A phase I trial using an HPV-16 E7 glutathione-S-transferase (GST) fusion protein in an Alum-based adjuvant has also been completed in cervical cancer patients. Generally these trials have been encouraging. The immunogen has been shown to be immunogenic and well tolerated and further trials designed to demonstrate efficacy are therefore warranted.

Additional developments in vaccine design seek to improve their efficacy. These include the use of new adjuvants but also more recently the use of immune modulatory genes in combination with the antigen of choice. For example chimeric protein fusions between E7 and the murine cytokine granulocyte macrophage colony-stimulating factor (GM-CSF) has been shown to enhance the immunogenicity of E7 in mice and a chimeric lysosomal-associated membrane protein 1 (LAMP-1) — E7 protein vaccinia recombinant has shown enhanced MHC class II presentation and shows significant anti-tumor activity in a murine E6/E7 tumor model. These studies are designed to invoke improved immune presentation of the antigen. GM-CSF is thought to induce differentiation and activation of antigen presenting cells (dendritic cells) at the site of innoculation (MHC class I pathway) and fusion with LAMP-1 will target antigen to endosomal and lysosomal compartments for processing and presentation by MHC class II molecules.

6.8.2 Prophylactic vaccines

Prophylactic protection against HPV infection is also is being investigated vigorously. There is very good and clear evidence that a strong neutralizing antibody (humoral) response can be effective in protecting animals from infection. CRPV L1 and L2 proteins, BPV-2 L1 (but not BPV-2 L2), and BPV-4 L2 bacterial fusion proteins have all been shown to be effective in protecting animals against challenge with the homologous animal virus.

An important advance in prophylactic vaccine design has been the development and use of papilloma virus-like particles (VLPs) [16]. Papillomavirus capsid proteins L1 and L2, or L1 alone will spontaneously assemble into a particle that is structurally and immunologically very similar to a natural virus particle. However, while VLPs are not exact immunological mimics of the natural virion both CRPV [17], and COPV and BPV-4 VLPs have all been shown to be protective in animal challenge studies. Human HPV-11 VLPs have also been generated and these have been shown to induce neutralizing antibody in rabbits and mice. Work with VLPs has shown that the strong neutralizing epitopes are conformationally dependent, and that neutralizing antibody may not be cross-reactive between HPV types. A broad spectrum prophylactic vaccine may therefore need to be multivalent. Phase I trials with human VLPs are now in progress.

Polynucleotide (DNA) vaccines are also very likely to be of value as human papillomavirus vaccines. While this technology is still being developed both neutralizing antibody and CTL responses have been invoked by DNA immunization in several experimental systems. In particular, immunization of cottontail rabbits with L2 and/or L1 expressing plasmids have recently been shown to protect against virus challenge [18]. DNA vaccination offers significant advantages over subunit, peptide and VLP approaches and whilst significant issues still need to be resolved it has considerable potential as a future treatment for human papillomavirus disease [19].

6.9 Conclusions

The human papillomaviruses comprise a broad group of closely related DNA viruses. While significant advances have been made in understanding viral replication, gene regulation, protein biochemistry, epidemiology and pathobiology important issues still remain. Understanding the immune recognition of HPV proteins by the host will impact upon vaccine design and both improved adjuvants and the use of co-stimulatory immune potentiating molecules will seek to improve vaccine efficacy. New targets for small molecule screening must await further investigations on the roles and biochemical functions of viral proteins and inparticular the E4 and E5 proteins.

The genotypic and phenotypic diversity with this group of viruses suggests that no single treatment against one or two genotypes is likely to be equally effective against them all. Consequently it is likely that effective treatment of HPV disease will make use of a number of different but complementary treatment strategies. Effective vaccines, small molecule inhibitors that are non-toxic, and specific inhibitors of viral replication and are urgently needed.

References

1. De Villiers, E.M. (1989) *J. Virol.,* **63**, 4898.
2. Brandsma, J.L. (1996) in *Papillomavirus Reviews: Current Research on Papillomaviruses*, (C. Lacey, ed.). Leeds University Press, Leeds.
3. Stoppler, M.C. Ching K., Stoppler H., Clancy K., Schlegel R. and Icenogle, J. (1996) *J.Virol.,* **70**: 6987.

4. Chow, L.T. and Broker T.R. (1994) *Intervirology,* **37**, 150.
5. *Virology*, 3rd Edn, (B.N. Fields, D.M. Knipe and P.M. Howley eds), Chapter 65, Vol. 2. Lippincott-Raven Press, p. 2045–2076.
6. Fuchs, P.G. and Pfister, H. (1996) in *Papillomarvirus Reviews: Current Research on Papillomarviruses* (C. Lacey, ed.). Leeds University Press, Leeds.
7. Cox, J.T. (1995) *Bailliere's Clinical Obstetrics and Gynaecology*, **9, 1**.
8. Ferenczy, A. (1995) *Am. J. Obstet. Gynecol.*, **172**, 1331.
9. Baker, G.E. and Tyring, S.K., (1997) *Dermatol. Clin.*, **15**, 331.
10. Rockley, P.F. and Tyring, S.K. (1995) *Pharmac. Ther.*, **65**, 265.
11. Phelps, W.C. and Alexander, K.A., (1995) *Ann. Intern. Med.* **123**, 368.
12. Plumpton, M., Sharp, N.A., Liddicoat, L.H., Remm, M., Tucker, D.O., Hughes, F.J., Russell, S.M. and Romanos, M.A. (1995) *BioTechnology*, **13**, 1210.
13. Tindle, R.W. and Frazer, I. (1995) *Exp. Opin. Invest. Drugs*, **4**, 783.
14. Selvakumar. R., Borenstein, L.A., Lin, Y.L. *et al.* (1995) *J.Virol.,* **69**, 602.
15. Van Driel, W.J., Ressing, M.E., Brandt, R.M.P., Toes, R.E.M., Fleuren, G.T., Trimbos, J.B., Kast, W.M. and Melief, C.J.M. (1996) *Annals of Medicine*, **28**, 471.
16. Kirnbauer, R. (1996) *Intervirology,* **39**, 54.
17. Jansen, K.U., Rosolowsky, M., Schultz, L.D., Markus, H.Z., Cook J.C., Donnelly, J.J., Martinez, D., Ellis, R.W. and Shaw, A.R. (1995) *Vaccine,* **13**, 1509.
18. Donnelly, J.J., Martinez, D., Jansen, K.U., Ellis, R.W., Montgomery, D.L. and Liu, M. (1996) *J. Inf. Diseases*, **713**, 314.
19. Ulmer, J.B., Donnelly, J.J. and Liu, M.A. (1996) *Curr. Opin. in Biotechnology*, **7**, 653.
20. Hildesheim, A. (1997) *J. Nat. Can. Inst.*, **89**, 752.

Chapter 7

Where next for antiviral therapies?

This chapter covers subject matter which we believe is not yet of sufficient significance or at a level of understanding to warrant individual chapters but may represent future growth areas for antiviral therapy, and adjunctive or novel regimens. Virus infections of organs such as the central nervous system (CNS) and the cardiovascular system are discussed, and we review briefly topics such as vaccination and emerging diseases. In the next few years it is likely that one or more of these subjects will become of considerably increased importance (*Table 7.1*).

Table 7.1: Viral targets and therapies

Virus	Indication	Therapeutic*
'Enzootic Viruses'	Haemorrhagic disease	sm, pv
Lassa (arena)	Haemorrhagic disease	sm, pv
Hantaan (bunya)	Haemorrhagic disease	sm, pv
Ebola (filo)	Haemorrhagic disease	sm, pv
HSV (herpes)	CNS (encephalitis	sm, pv
Measles (paramyxo)	CNS	pv
Rabies (rhabdo)	CNS	tv
Polio (picorna)	CNS	pv
Rubella (toga)	CNS	pv
Borna (unclassified)	CNS	pv
HIV (retro)	CNS (dementia)	sm, tv
Coxsackie (picorna)	Cardiovascular	sm, tv
HCMV (herpes)	Cardiovascular (restenosis)	sm, pv, tv
HCV (flavir)	Cardiovascular	sm, pv, tv, it
HPV (papilloma)	Epithelial neoplasia	sm, pv, tv
RSV (paramyxo)	Asthma, COPD	sm, pv, it
Influenza (orthomyxo)	Asthma, COPD	sm, pv, tv
HRV (picorna)	Asthma, COPD	sm, it
Paraflu 3 (paramyxo)	Asthma, COPD	sm, pv, tv

* sm = small molecule; pv = prophylactic vaccine; tv = therapeutic vaccine; it = immunotherapy.

7.1 Future targets

7.1.1 Emerging diseases

History has taught us that the relationship between the human population and viruses (and other pathogens) is a fluid one and there are numerous examples of the emergence of infections which have had profound consequences. Moreover, it is probable that the incidence of viral emergence is accelerating as a consequence of the changing human life-style and ever increasing disruption of the global environment. The reasons underlying this trend are many fold and include: (1) the huge increase in the human population or host pool; (2) the dramatically increased rate and extent of travel with concomitant potential for rapid dissemination; (3) the disruption of natural ecosystems with increased exposure of humans to previously 'isolated' sources of infection; (4) the accidental transfer and introduction of virus vectoring arthropods to new parts of the world, and (5) improved detection and isolation of new viruses.

Emerging viruses pose particularly difficult problems to health control authorities since, by their very nature, they have the potential for serious impact on public health that is difficult to predict. How much effort and expenditure should be lavished on a newly described virus disease which at one extreme may only infect a few individuals or at the other may cause an international pandemic? Quarantine and standard hygienic measures are relatively inexpensive to implement and would be set in place as a matter of routine if monitoring procedures were sufficiently good to warn international health authorities of a possible important infectious disease risk. If these measures fail the development of vaccines and drugs would be the next response along with increased transmission control measures such as vector control. A practical constraint on this scenario is the economic one since developing drugs and vaccines is a slow, expensive and uncertain exercise. This is evidenced by the AIDS situation in which, despite huge investment, the prospects of an effective vaccine are as far away as ever (see below). In addition despite recent advances which have identified effective drug combination therapies, there is no evidence as yet as to a curative treatment. Furthermore, most emerging viruses appear in developing countries with limited health budgets.

A dramatic illustration of the effects that emergent viruses can have is provided by the pandemics of influenza infection that have arisen during this century and have been responsible for the loss of millions of lives. Each has been caused by a new virus which has arisen through reassortment of avian and human virus gene segments, almost certainly in an intermediate host (pig). The resulting new viruses possessed totally new antigenic characteristics and so could spread unchecked through an immunologically naïve population, with devastating results. Of course, it is now possible to produce vaccines against new influenza viruses relatively rapidly but this almost certainly lags behind the spread of disease which can circumnavigate the globe in months. A current example is the new influenza A variant H5N1, to which there is no pre-existing immunity and which appears to been transmitted from domesticated fowl. It would seem prudent, therefore to augment the armaments against influenza with drug therapies as well as vaccines. There are now two drugs which have significant activity against most influenza viruses and so, to a limited extent, fulfil the aspirations of developing drugs which are effective against a range of potential emergent viruses. These are ramantidine and zanamivir, which were discussed in Chapter 4, and both would be effective against the H5N1 variant although zanamivir is not yet licensed.

Another example of a virus that is thought to have emerged from an animal host is HIV. In this case there is a clear genetic similarity between HIV-2 and a retrovirus of monkeys (sooty monkey virus). It is not clear what factors led to the transmission of this agent to humans or its spread beyond a limited number of individuals to become a world-wide problem. It is also not clear as to the identity of a similar animal virus progenitor for HIV-1.

One group of agents commonly classified as emerging viruses are enzootic RNA viruses and there are a number of theoretic rationalizations of why this should be so. Also, most are responsible for hemorrhagic disease symptoms. Given the costs of discovering and developing drugs, the most economically effective route to producing medicines for these infections would be to concentrate on 'generic' products effective against a wide range of viruses, e.g. by inhibiting common features such as the dependence on an RNA-dependent RNA polymerase for replication, or by treating common features of the induced pathology. Whether or not such 'windows of opportunity' for cross-reactive disease intervention therapy actually exist is, of course, unknown but the potential strategic value of drugs fulfilling this requirement in the face of an explosive emergent disease would be great indeed.

As stated above, most emerging viruses result from the spill over of infection from one animal reservoir into another, usually following environmental disturbance. Examples are Lassa fever, which is an asymptomatic virus of forest rodents in Africa but which can cause disease with very high mortality in humans. A similar scenario is seen with Hanta viruses in Asia, several Arenaviruses in South America and, recently another Hantavirus, Sin Nombre virus, in North America. A particularly alarming virus, Ebola, also emerges periodically from central African forests to produce small, but deadly outbreaks of disease. Despite considerable effort, the natural host of the virus has not been identified as yet. The disease has been transmitted out of Africa with infected batches of monkeys and one strain appeared to be transmissible by aerosol. Fortunately, this strain did not appear to be able to infect humans, but the incident illustrates the potential for serious epidemic dispersion of new and serious disease. Of course, viruses are adapted, in general, to particular host species and are unlikely to immediately assume a natural balance with a new host (humans for example). However, this stabilization process, may involve dramatic effects on the new host, as evidenced by the introduction of Myxoma virus to European rabbit populations.

The emergence of hepatitis C virus as a major human pathogen is, at least in part, due to the development of diagnostic techniques. Most infections appears to be benign for many years and serious disease frequently develops long after initial infection. Clearly, in such a situation epidemiological analysis based on symptomology is bound to be highly inaccurate.

Future scenarios which could lead to an emerging virus are at present being discussed and investigated. For example concern over transmission of viruses from a natural porcine host into humans is one of the major concerns relating to organ transplants from transgenic pigs. Rapid rejection of transplanted pig organs occurs due to the recognition of terminal sugar residues, such as α1–3 galactose, on the donor organs by human antibodies. Transgenic pigs have a new sugar transferase (fucosyl α1–2) and this competes with α1–3 galactosyl transferase for terminal glycosylation of proteins. These transgenic animals are essentially deleted for the α1–3 galactosyl transferase, as are humans naturally, so that these organs are no longer rejected on this basis by human recipients. However, recent studies have identified a number of endogenous porcine retroviruses in these organs. As well as being transferred within the organ, these retroviruses may be produced within humans without the α1–3 galactose residue on its envelope, thus rendering the virus stable in human serum. It has long been thought that retroviruses whether C-type, lenti or foamy etc., produced from lower primates, as well as other animals and birds, would not cross the species barrier into human because of their instability in human serum, due to complement inactivation. As compliment inactivation is also mediated by antibody recognition of α1–3 galactose, then porcine retroviruses released from transgenic pigs or from their transplanted organs would be substantially more stable in human blood and have greater opportunity to infect humans. Clearly, there are enough examples in nature of the species barrier being crossed into man without man himself providing further opportunities, and so some considerable thought is needed on the risks and benefits of transplanting organs from these transgenic animals. Another such example is seen when one considers the spread of feline parvo virus to the dog population. When this emergent virus infects a young dog it may lead to a severe disease and death. Detailed comparisons have shown that a single nucleotide change in the feline parvo virus was sufficient to alter its species tropism with dramatic effect. One can only speculate if a similar 'minor' change could lead to this virus infecting humans. Finally it is clear with the eradication of smallpox virus that monkeypox virus had been (and still is) infecting humans with a resulting mortality rate similar to that of the major, highly virulent strain of smallpox. Fortunately this virus can only spread from monkey to humans by intimate contact and not from human to human. Once again, however, if this agent was to adapt to the human environment its spread in the unprotected population could have serious consequences.

7.1.2 Viruses and the CNS

The pathological connection between viruses and the CNS is a varied one. In some cases infection by a given virus precedes a clear disease association with marked sequalae while others have a more chronic progression with symptoms which are not obviously caused by virus infection. For example, herpesviruses, paramyxoviruses (measles virus and canine distemper virus) and retroviruses have been suggested to have a potential role in multiple sclerosis.

There are a number of viruses which have the cells of the CNS as their principle site of replication. The best example of this is rabies virus. After infection the virus is thought to replicate in local muscle tissue before it invades the peripheral nervous system. After infection of the peripheral nerves it travels up the axons at a rate of 3 mm h^{-1} and once the virus has entered the brain it spreads to form a widespread disseminated disease. There is believed to be a strong immune pathological basis in the damage caused by rabies virus infection. Also there are results that show that the ability of the rabies virus to fuse cell membranes is associated with pathogenicity although the mechanism is unclear.

The number of people treated each year for potential rabies infection is still large (ca. 1 million) with some 50 000 deaths in people not treated. Fortunately although there are no small molecules with anti-rabies activity, the length of the incubation period from bite to CNS involvement allows the use of a vaccine to raise the immune response. This coupled with good wound management is a highly effective therapy.

Other viruses can infect and cause disease in several tissue types including the CNS. Common examples of these viruses include herpes simplex virus and polio although this list could be extended to include VZV, HCMV, HIV, influenza virus and others. In the case of polio virus, infection is usually limited to the gastrointestinal tract and only about 1% of infections result in recognized clinical symptoms. The most common form of recognized disease caused by polio virus is abortive poliomyelitis which has 'flu' like symptoms with headache, fever, sore throat etc. The prognosis of such infections is good. Nonparalytic poliomyelitis has the same symptoms as abortive but also has associated back pain. In young children a fourth type of polio virus-induced illness can arise — paralytic poliomyelitis. In this case infection of the CNS causes flaccid paralysis resulting from lower motor neurone damage. The amount of damage varies from case to case and recovery takes up to 6 months. It is during intracellular replication of virus in some nerve cells that damage is caused. Virus replication leads to an inflammatory response which culminates in drastic consequences such as lifelong residual paralysis or death. The development of very effective vaccines for polio have dramatically reduced the frequency of CNS disease.

HSV infection of the CNS causes an encephalitis which in the absence of therapy may lead to death in 50% of cases. In those patients that resolve their infection some are left with severe neurological impairment. The discovery of aciclovir had a major impact on the outcome of herpes virus associated encephalitis with survival rates increasing significantly (see Chapter 2).

In the case of HIV infection, penetration of the CNS may cause disease by a number of mechanisms; either by releasing cytokines from infected microglial (macrophage) cells; direct cell destruction of key cells or abnormal immune response to HIV proteins. It is also possible that infection of the CNS by HIV is associated with the presence of a number of AIDS associated co-factors such as JC virus, HCMV or EBV which by themselves or in association with HIV cause CNS disease. Many HIV infected people report CNS problems including difficulties with balance, weakness, pain and behavioral changes. In a number of extreme cases AIDS-associated dementia may occur with a survival time of some 6 months to 1 year. There is good evidence that anti-retroviral therapy can prevent HIV-associated CNS disease. As AZT has been shown to penetrate the blood–brain barrier it is also possible that the use of this compound may also have a direct anti-HIV effect in the CNS. For other anti-HIV agents the ability to penetrate the blood–brain barrier is an important property which may influence its utility, and new compounds are in development with such characteristics (see Chapter 3).

Influenza virus infection causes significant CNS disease. These include drowsiness and irritability through to coma. However, in most cases these symptoms are thought to be caused by the nonspecific effects of high temperature and fever caused by influenza virus infection. In some cases influenza is thought to cause an encephalopathy or post-encephalitic disease, but both conditions are rare and in most cases there is little evidence for virus in the CNS.

There is little evidence that measles virus has any neurotropic properties. However, in rare cases so-called abortive replication of measles virus in the CNS may cause subacute sclerosing panencephalitis (SSPE). The incubation period from infection to disease symptoms is over 7 years. The mechanism of disease formation is not clear with some evidence of differences in the genotype of the virus found in the CNS while other studies suggest that the immune response of the patient is a factor. With the widespread use of measles vaccine it will be interesting to see if the incidence of SSPE decreases in the future.

Another aspect of virus-associated CNS disease involves the infection of the unborn fetus. Examples of such agents include rubella and cytomegalovirus. While rare, such infections of the fetus can be catastrophic, resulting in sequalae including moderate to severe learning difficulties and deafness. The consequence of infection by rubella virus *in utero* can be prevented by vaccination of the potential mother during childhood and by boosting the immune response of females at puberty or before pregnancy occurs. In the case of HCMV in the US alone some 40 000 children are born each year with congenital infection. The consequence of this infection include hearing loss, HCMV is considered to be a major cause of hearing loss and learning difficulties in children. Primary infection of the mother is the most common cause of infection with between 30 and 50% transmission to the fetus. Transmission due to a reccurrence is much lower. This suggests that the immune response of the mother may limit spread of the virus to the fetus. Unfortunately there is no current vaccine for HCMV and no licensed drug for treatment of children.

Links between virus infections and neurological aberrations continue to emerge, even for conditions well defined in terms of neurological involvement that have not been traditionally associated with virus infection. For example, there has been a recent study showing a potential association between herpes simplex virus infection and Alzheimer's disease. As yet the association has not been formally proven and the mechanism by which HSV may cause or trigger Alzheimer's is not clear. If proven prophylactic antiviral therapy or vaccination may be useful for prevention or treatment of Alzheimer's disease. There are also some findings that link Borna virus to some human psychiatric disorders. Borna virus is a negative single-stranded RNA virus which may infect a wide variety of animals including horses, sheep, cattle and domestic animals such as the cat. In several of these species infection by Borna virus is clearly associated with neurological sequalae including learning difficulties, insomnia and behavior changes such as aggression. Virus is found in the brains of infected animals and it is thought that the disease is caused by an inflammatory response mediated by $CD8^+$ T cells. There are clear seroepidemiological data that show that humans are infected by Borna and some studies suggest that there is an increase in seroprevalence in patients with neurological conditions such as schizophrenia and depression. It is difficult to envisage antiviral therapy for Borna virus infection as there are few apparent symptoms associated with primary infection in humans. However, if proven there would be a clear opportunity for a vaccine to prevent or reduce the severity of Borna virus infection and the subsequent neurological diseases.

7.1.3 Other aetiologies

Heart and muscle disease.   Coxsackie B virus has strong links with myocardial disease. Viral association with disease has been shown in a number of different studies, both autopsy tissue colocalization studies, and in adults and children who subsequently develop disease, the recent infection rates have been shown to be in the range 25–40%. Nonhuman primates artificially infected with coxsackie B have been shown to develop heart disease that is exacerbated by both exercise and a range of other factors which in humans are also known to increase the risk of compromising myocardial function. The underlying cause for the pathology is not clear but inflammatory responses to infected heart tissue imply an immunopathological basis.

Associations between heart muscle disease and infection have been established for HCMV. HCMV is a herpesvirus and virus proteins and nucleic acid can be detected in heart muscle and arterial endothelial cells. HCMV can establish a latent infection and genomic copies and viral transcripts have been detected in the smooth muscle cell layer of the large arteries and heart tissue of seropositive patients although it is not clear as to whether HCMV is truly latent in these cells. It is suggested that stimulation of HCMV in these tissues (perhaps as a result of tissue damage during operative procedures) may contribute both to atherosclerosis and to restenosis following angioplasty. Lesions from restenosis patients have been shown to contain transcripts from the HCMV immediate-early (IE) gene region and the *IE84* gene which may be expressed from these IE sequences has recently been shown to bind and inhibit the activity of the tumor-suppressor protein p53. In this way HCMV could promote smooth muscle cell proliferation and invoke a pathogenic cascade [2].

The link between HCMV and both restenosis and atherosclerosis remains unproven but the established pathobiology of this virus and the mechanistic link recently identified justifies further investigation. If these are proven then existing antiviral chemotherapeutic agents or vaccines could be used in disease management. However, before such approaches could be used a clear understanding of the relationship between HCMV and these diseases would need to be established. For example, if HCMV is already present in tissues before reactivation then disease could be triggered without virus replication and therefore standard antiviral agents would not be of use for treatment of such conditions. They may be of use prophylactically, however, and a more sensible approach may be to reduce or even prevent the burden of HCMV in these tissues by prophylactic vaccination.

A number of other viruses have also been linked to heart disease. HIV infection has been associated with cardiomyopathy and myocarditis in adults. This is more common in infected children but in both cases the pathogenic mechanisms are unclear. Infection of heart tissue also occurs during infection with Mumps virus. Rarely fatal and usually asymptomatic these infections can result in abnormal functioning of heart muscle and this probably reflects mild pericarditis and/or myocarditis. More recently abundant genomic copies of hepatitis C virus have been detected in patients with cardiomyopathy and myocarditis, and isolated cases of mycocarditis following retrovirus infection have been reported. However, in both cases a direct link between viral infection and pathology is speculative and remains unproved.

Postviral fatigue syndrome.   A condition known as postviral fatigue syndrome has been recognized for several decades but considerable controversy still surrounds this difficult area of medicine and many still believe the condition to be a psychosomatic illness. However, there are now many documented cases of the syndrome in individuals who have no prior history of psychosomatic disorders and the evidence is compelling that at least in some people the disease has an underlying physical cause. The syndrome is more commonly known today as ME (myalgic encephalomyelitis) although even this name is inappropriate since so far there is no evidence for pathology in the nervous system. The symptoms include chronic tiredness and severe muscle weakness, sometimes accompanied by headaches and depression, and they can persist for months or years. It is still an open question whether this disease has an underlying virus aetiology. It is not uncommon for viruses to be proposed as aetiological agents of a disease when no other cause can be found, and with ME several viruses from diverse families have been suggested. The front runners are Epstein–Barr virus and the enterovirus, coxsackie B3, but with other possible candidates such as human herpesvirus-6 and influenza. Much more work will be required to determine whether these associated virus infections have a causative role in the disease and whether they provide us with therapeutic opportunities.

Chronic respiratory disease.   There is little doubt that viral infections contribute to asthma exacerbations, with initial reports appearing in 1976 on the role of human rhinovirus (HRV) and influenza virus (Flu). However, the best studies to date are those performed in Southampton into the role of respiratory viruses in childhood asthma, which showed that viruses were associated with 77% of asthma exacerbations and that rhinoviruses represented the most common agent, followed by coronaviruses (CV). Recent data from the same laboratories suggest that the viral prevalence is about the same in exacerbations of adult asthma, and appears to reflects the circulating levels of all respiratory viruses, including HRV, CV, RSV, Flu and parainfluenza (see Chapter 4). As asthma is in part due to airway hypersensitivity, then agents, such as Flu and HRV, which are known to cause hyperreactivity in the lower respiratory tract following infection of the upper respiratory tract were obvious candidates. Part of the hyper-responsiveness induced by Flu appears to be the result of direct desquamation of the airway epithelia, and also by alterations in function of the M2 muscarinic receptor as a result of the viral neuraminidase enzyme cleaving sialic acid from the receptor proteins. For HRV, and RSV, many of the effects on asthma appear to mediated by the cytokines produced from infected airway epithelia which recruit activated eosinophils into the mucosa of the airways. Long residence times of activated eosinopils are defining characteristics of asthma, and virus may extend such residence times further. Other mechanisms, including stimulation of IgE, histamine and prostaglandin release from mast cells (basophils) as an indirect result of virus (HRV, Flu, RSV etc) infection clearly also contributes to disease [3].

Chronic obstructive pulmonary disease (COPD), such as emphysema and chronic bronchitis, are increasingly seen in our aging population, and again there is good evidence to suggest a role for viral pathogens [4]. Like asthma, this disease is partly driven by infiltration of leukocytes, but in the case of COPD the cell types are predominantly neutrophils. Again recruitment and activation of neutrophils would result from the immunopathology associated with HRV- and RSV infection of airway epithelia and lung macrophages (IL-8 and TNF-α production), and although studies in 1980 suggested that 18% of COPD exacerbations were associated with viral infections of the respiratory tract, the particular viruses associated with specific manifestations of COPD remain to be elucidated.

Finally, there are some suggestions that RSV, as the major viral pathogen of new-born babies, may actually cause subsequent wheeze and asthma, particularly in children with a genetic predisposition to atopy. This hypothesis again relates to the unusual T_h2 skewed immunopathology of RSV, and suggests that the development of the T_h1 helper T cell population post-partum is suppressed or prevented by RSV infection. A key study would be to establish the number of children born of atopic parents who developed asthma, and whether RSV infection, which has a well-defined season of about four to five winter months, influenced this.

7.2 Vaccines and immunomodulators

7.2.1 Viruses for which the development of vaccines is difficult

HIV.   It has long been apparent that the best vaccinations are those that give rise to a level of immunity as close as possible to that raised by the infectious agent itself. This is particularly true for HIV where not only is it desirable to mount both cell- mediated and humoral immunity, but a high level of mucosal immunity may also prove to be necessary for an effective preventative vaccine. While this may well be feasible for HIV and the at-risk populations can be clearly identified, the prospects for widespread uptake of a targeted prophylactic vaccination program are not expected to be particularly high. Therefore, we are left to ponder how to generate a therapeutic vaccine against HIV given that the nature of the disease caused by HIV is a generalized immune dysfunction. In addition, the virus itself presents some unique problems. Firstly, the virus replicates and kills key effector cells of the immune system including macrophages and helper T cells. Secondly, the virus life cycle incorporates a proviral stage whereby the pathogen can be immunologically silent. Thirdly, the virus may be present in compartments, such as the peripheral and CNS, that are not usually accessible to the immune system. Finally, as full-blown AIDS develops from the various precursor stages, the loss of helper T cells means that even immunity to previously harmless 'endogenous' bacterial and fungal pathogens is lost. These problems may be insurmountable, but recent success with vaccination of chimpanzees against SIV suggests that some renewed effort in this area may be appropriate.

One way to view a therapeutic vaccine to HIV is as an adjunctive to anti-retroviral combination therapies. As alluded to in Chapter 3, the latest triple and quadruple drug combinations have successfully lowered plasma and certain cell-associated HIV levels over long periods. It seems reasonable to treat those patients with a prospective HIV vaccine and then monitor the efficacy by release from retroviral therapy. It is known that release from triple therapy results in a rapid increase in plasma levels of HIV; an effective vaccine may prevent this rebound. The problem of immunologically silent provirus may be overcome by short-term treatment with IL-2 during vaccination. In this situation, IL-2 would stimulate transcription of the provirus eventually leading to *de novo* protein production, and although protease anti-retroviral therapy would prevent release of HIV, appearance of gp160 or its gp120/gp41 products on the surface of macrophages would not be affected. In addition, MHC class I presentation of gag-, pol- and env-related peptides would not, theoretically, be affected by any of the antiviral therapies. In addition, secreted gp120 may also raise some humoral immunity, and the presence of IL-2 would also enhance cell-mediated immunity to both *de novo* antigens and vaccine antigens. This type of IL-2 immune therapy could have enhanced value since it has been shown that many proviruses are defective for virion production (some 90% of proviruses!), but most these viruses would still produce some form of viral antigen in response to transcriptional activation. The danger may be that over-expression of viral antigens on dendritic cells could contribute to the loss of lymph node architecture that is part of HIV immunopathogenesis, but much of this pathogenesis occurs in the late stages of disease and may be avoided with an almost intact immune system

The question still remains as to which antigens should be used and how these antigens should be delivered. There is some thought that many of the gp160/gp120 vaccines failed because the recombinant protein was produced in monomeric form, whereas the natural target for ADCC and humoral immunity appears to be the gp160/gp120 trimer. New trimeric gp120 may be a suitable subunit vaccine. In order that mucosal immunity be raised, there is some debate around using specialized delivery vectors, such as Venezuelan equine encephalitis virus, or using combinations of DNA vaccines with adenovirus delivered endogenous expression. Of course, as vaccination regimes become more exotic, the costs and complexities may become prohibitive to widespread vaccinations particularly in developing countries. In this latter scenario, the 'gene guns' being developed by several biotechnology companies may make widespread DNA vaccinations effective and economically viable. Finally, many groups are developing defective HIV as vehicles for antigen delivery; however, increasing evidence of recombination in HIV giving rise to chimeric cross-clade viruses may mean some thought needs to be given to the nature of the defect in the HIV vehicle. In addition, recombination probably means that vaccines should be multivalent and incorporate epitopes in gag and/or env that are clade specific.

Paradoxically, it is the success of antiviral therapy that offers hope for the development of HIV vaccines.

HCV. Hepatitis C virus provides another example of an infection against which there is little possibility for the development of an effective prophylactic vaccine in the foreseeable future. The virus shows a great propensity for sequence variation, especially in regions thought to represent important antigenic features. In this respect it resembles HIV and it is likely that the problems attendant on the development of an anti-HIV vaccine will apply equally to HCV. In addition, it has been shown that chimpanzees that have recovered from HCV infection are completely susceptible to infection with the same virus inoculum, which casts doubt on the concept that effective immunity can be induced. Moreover, most infections initiate a long-term, possibly lifelong, chronic state which is responsible for ultimate serious liver disease. Therefore, there will continue to be a great number of patients in need of therapeutic benefit even if an effective vaccine were developed and widely used tomorrow.

Common cold (rhinoviruses). Many of us experience at least one cold of varying severity every year, and unless this occurs during the winter peaks of viruses such as respiratory syncytial virus or influenza, it is most likely caused by a rhinovirus. Even in middle age we still get infected by rhinoviruses. The reason for this is that there are more than 100 serologically different types of HRV and an antibody response to one virus does not protect against subsequent infection by a different serotype. For this same reason, development of a vaccine against rhino-viruses is very unlikely. There is so much variation among the immunologically dominant sites in the major capsid proteins of HRV (VP1-VP4) that cross-neutral-izing antibodies have not been identified. Although the replicative enzymes of HRV, such as the 3C protease or the 3D polymerase, are highly conserved, they are presented as epitope fragments either very poorly or very rarely, so that there is only ever a weak immune response. Indeed, the highly conserved nature of these proteins would suggest little or no immune selection, but the sequence conservation makes the possibility of a small-molecule pan-rhinovirus therapeutic likely.

RSV.   Respiratory syncytial viruses cause a flu-like upper respiratory tract infection in many healthy children which is self limited and rarely life-threatening. Infection of adults leads generally to less severe symptoms. Conversely, in the immunocompromised or the elderly, RSV-associated pneumonitis and pneumonia are a source of great morbidity and considerable mortality. However, it is in very young infants, particularly premature babies, that RSV bronchiolitis and pneumonia are responsible for a great number of hospitalizations that frequently end in death. It is this latter population that is the key target for antiviral therapy, as discussed in Chapter 4, and has been the test population for vaccine trials in the past. One such vaccine, based upon formalin-inactivated RSV, resulted in enhanced disease in vaccinated children following subsequent natural infections, and resulted in hospitalization of 100% of the vaccinees in many trial centers in the early 1970s. The findings that the formalin-inactivated RSV vaccine enhanced disease has resulted in a very slow cautious approach to development of subsequent vaccines. The recent recognition of the roles of T_h1/T_h2 population improved our understanding of T helper cells and their associated cytokine profiles, and have provided possible reasons for the complications of the formalin-inactivated vaccine and allowed more rational development of subunit or attenuated RSV vaccines.

Experiments with individual surface glycoproteins of RSV, F and G have shown that F induces T_h1 cytokines, whereas G is responsible for the induction of T_h2 cytokines. Formalin has since been shown to inactivate F, thus suppressing T_h1 cytokine production, but has little or no effect on G. Thus the formalin-inactivated vaccine was akin to inoculating babies with purified G or an allergen, stimulating a T_h2 response that was subsequently enhanced by natural infection to give bronchiolitis in 100% of cases. Armed with this understanding it is clear that F represents the best subunit vaccine candidate, whereas an attenuated vaccine with functional F, in the presence of G, probably also represents a safe approach. By a quirk of nature, F is considerably less variable among clinical isolates of RSV than G, and so with the benefit of hindsight, F would appear to be the best subunit vaccine. A number of subunit and other vaccines for RSV are in trial and development and may prove to be effective. If so then the impact of RSV disease in at risk populations may be reduced.

7.2.2 Therapeutic vaccines

Some of the notable successes in the management of viral disease have been with vaccines. Among these are measles, mumps, rubella, polio and smallpox. Hepatitis A and hepatitis B vaccines and a chickenpox vaccine are also now available. However, all of these vaccines are used prophylactically and one of the challenges of viral vaccine development is the generation of effective vaccines that have therapeutic utility and which therefore can be used to manage persistent viral infections.

The clinical outcome of any infection reflects the balance between the ability of the pathogen to persist and spread and the ability of the host immune response to control and eliminate the infection. In most viral infections the progress of the disease is rapid and the symptoms are of an acute nature. Typically, a virus establishes infection rapidly in order to replicate and shed sufficient progeny to ensure further spread before the host immune response is sufficient to eliminate or at least effectively control the infection. The clinical consequences will obviously be influenced by the rate of damage induction by the virus on the one hand and the speed with which the immune response can be mounted on the other. Drugs which may help to damp down the rate of viral replication during the induction phase of the immune response, and thus reduce symptoms, are clearly desirable but therapeutic vaccines are unlikely to have a role in this situation. With chronic infections, however, there is a great potential for the development of therapeutic vaccines. However, targeting chronic viral infection with a vaccine in order to invoke a host immune response that eliminates the reservoir of virus presents a number of obstacles. It has recently become clear that viruses that have evolved to persist in the host have developed a battery of evasive tactics in order to avoid detection and elimination by the immune system. The herpesviruses appear to be masters of immune evasion. They are known to establish lifelong latent infections in sites that are immunologically privileged (e.g. HSV in the peripheral nervous system), and encode a number of gene products which together block viral antigen presentation to the immune system. They have also been shown to encode mimics of cell surface immune markers, mimics of immune regulatory molecules (chemokines and cytokines), and decoy immune regulatory receptor molecules [5].

Chronic infections, by definition represent a failure of the host immune system to eliminate the pathogen, even if it is sufficient to prevent rampant spread of infection. The ability to up-regulate the natural response to a sufficient level to eliminate infection is probably the most hopeful route to truly curative treatments of chronic viral infections. The cell-mediated response of the immune system is thought to be the most important arm for the elimination of ongoing virus infection. In order to determine the most effective way to produce a potential therapeutic vaccine it is first important to determine the crucial T cell epitopes responsible for effective recognition by immune cells and to understand of the best way to present them to the host for maximum response.

One possible approach is a therapeutic regimen which combines the use of antiviral drugs and vaccines, as discussed for HIV vaccinations (7.2.1). With hepatitis B and C chronic infections the outcome of interferon treatment, which at least in part exerts its effects by immunomodulation, is better when the rate of virus replication is least. In the case of HBV similar strategies may emerge with agents such as lamivudine.

An obvious concern relating to the induction of powerful cell-mediated responses is that this may be akin to an autoimmune response, resulting in massive destruction of infected host tissue. Recent experiments with transgenic animals designed to address this issue have shown, however, that effective control of HBV expression can be achieved by immune T cells without the destruction of infected cells. This is mediated by cytokines produced by the T cells and provides more encouragement for optimism regarding the future potential of therapeutic vaccine approaches.

In order to invoke an immune response that clears a persistent viral infection potent T-cell responses must be induced against viral antigens. Therapeutic vaccine strategies have therefore sought to achieve this. Consequently peptide vaccines using amino acid sequences containing established T-cell epitopes to viral antigens have been identified and developed. These are being used in conjunction with existing and novel new adjuvants and it is hoped that both components will together generate a sufficiently strong response to clear infection. Whole protein vaccines (subunit vaccine) comprising purified viral proteins known to contain a range of T-cell (and B-cell) epitopes are also being tested. Adjuvants are again a feature of these candidate viral vaccines. Subunit vaccines have been developed using HSV proteins and while these have looked encouraging in animal models the results in clinical trials of a subunit HSV vaccine has proven disappointing.

Another approach is the use of replication defective/disabled viruses, e.g. for HSV, influenza and RSV. Such candidate vaccines may offer advantage because they deliver to the host the full complement of viral proteins for presentation to the host immune system. Partial replication of the virus further facilitates generation of a good immune response since following infection of host cells viral proteins synthesized inside the cell will engage the MHC class I pathway of antigen presentation. This should in turn invoke a strong cytotoxic T-cell (CTL) response. One of the limitations of this approach is to find the correct balance between disabling the ability of the virus to replicate (attenuation), while allowing sufficient expression of viral proteins for good antigen presentation. Over attenuation can lead to poor immune responses while under-attenuation can lead to adverse reactions in the vaccinee. An elegant system that appears to combine the required aspects of immunity and safety is the recently developed herpes simplex virus DISC (disabled infectious single cycle) system. HSV virus that is deleted in the glycoprotein H gene (*gH*) replicates and generates infectious virions only in cells that can provide (complement) the deleted *gH* gene in *trans*. In noncomplementing cells in the host the gH null virus replicates fully in uninfected cells and releases gH null virions which bud from the cell but cannot then re-infect new cells. This feature allows full replication and synthesis of all viral genes products in the hosts cells while restricting viral dissemination to a single cycle. Guinea-pig animal studies have shown that HSV DISC can significantly reduce recurrent disease [6]. HSV DISC is currently in clinical trials for treatment of recurrent genital herpes (see Chapter 2).

Finally, a new technology which offers significant advantage over proteinaceous and peptide vaccines is the development of candidate naked DNA vaccines. They offer significant cost savings and speed of development and while safety (genomic integration) remains a long-term concern it is likely that naked DNA vaccines will herald a new age in vaccines. The use of genes that encode T cell epitopes for example non-structural proteins will be used in therapeutic naked DNA vaccines.

7.2.3 Cytokines as therapeutics

The rise of biotechnology has made it relatively simple to obtain large quantities of recombinant cytokines for administration as therapeutics, either in their own right or as adjunctives to small molecule antivirals, or vaccines. However, there is reason to remember traditional means of producing therapeutic immunomodulators; the lymphoblastoid cell-produced family of IFN-α (Wellferon) apparently outperforms some *E.coli*-produced recombinant INF-α in some clinical trails with HBV and HCV sufferers.

HBV. A transgenic model of HBV disease has thrown up some observations which suggest that it may be possible to clear HBV from infected livers, using IFN-γ and TNF-α, without killing the hepatocytes that carry the virus. It was generally thought that viral clearance was mediated by recognition and killing of virus infected cells by cytotoxic T cells (CTLs) activated by viral antigens. However, adoptive transfer of CTLs, primed beforehand *in vitro* with HBV-derived peptides, resulted in the loss of viral DNA and RNA from many more hepatocytes than those that could have been killed directly. In addition, there was an inflammatory influx of other effector cells (polymorphs and leukocytes), and so there appeared to be a soluble mediator released by the CTLs. These mediators were shown to be IFN-γ and TNF-α. Further experiments, showing that IL-12 enhanced viral clearance, suggested that IFN-γ and TNF-α released from helper T-cells are also involved in this process and that a cocktail of IL-12 plus IFN-γ and TNF-α could be the preferred regimen. This so-called 'non-cytolytic clearance' of HBV would be an extremely valuable alternative to current therapies, and studies are underway to see if the same mechanisms could be used to clear other chronic viral infections such as HCV and HPV.

RSV. It has long been recognized from studying the nasal secretions of infected babies, and also experimentation in small animal models, that RSV disease is caused to large extent by an underlying immunopathology. The contents of nasal secretions, containing histamines, prostaglandins and other allergen response factors derived from eosinophils, and the role of CD4$^+$ helper cells in mouse disease pathology, suggest that infection with RSV induces a high levels of T$_h$2 cytokines (see Chapter 3). In cell culture, T$_h$2 cytokines such as IL-6 and IL-8 are released from RSV infected respiratory airways epithelial cells and also lung (alveolar) macrophages, and it is known that chemokines (RANTES) and pro-inflammatory cytokines (TNF-α) are also released. The role of IL-8 and RANTES in eosinophil recruitment is well documented, and is discussed above in the context of chronic respiratory disease, but recent data suggest that RSV immunopathology can be reversed in mice by antibodies to IL-5, an eosinophil activating cytokine; this raises the possibility that the same may be true in man. Clearly, reversing the severity of RSV infection in babies using local (inhaled) delivery of cytokine antagonists or agonists may be feasible since the 'window of opportunity' to inhibit RSV replication is small whereas the immunopathology is prolonged.

HIV.   As discussed in Chapter 3, the identification of the HIV co-receptors as primarily CCKR5 on macrophages, and CXCR4 on T cells, and the observation that the switch in replication levels associated with the more virulent syncytium inducing (SI) phenotype is associated with a switch from CCKR5 to CXCR4, suggests that virus inhibition chemokine antagonists could be feasible. Studies have shown that horizontally transmitted HIV tends to enter the new host via cells of the macrophage lineage, and so CCKR5 antagonists may well prevent transmission of the virus. A chemically modified version of recombinant (met)RANTES, called AOP-RANTES, was shown to be a potent antagonist of natural RANTES and to suppress HIV infection of macrophages and peripheral blood lymphocytes. However, recent data showing that people who were homozygous for the $\Delta 32$ mutation, which inactivates CCKR5, could none the less still become infected upon exposure to HIV, suggests that blocking transmission of macrophage tropic HIV may not be sufficient. Furthermore, the complexity of the interaction of the virus with CCKR5 suggests that small molecule inhibitors with the potency of AOP-RANTES may be hard to find. If the virus that infects people via a CCKR5-independent route is an SI variant with other chemokine co-receptor utilization, then the prospects of developing a chemokine antagonist as a viral inhibitor are even less likely since these variants appear, in cell culture at least, to use the CCR3 and CCR2 chemokine receptors, in addition to CXCR4. Although the theory appears good, in practice chemokine antagonists may not offer alternative HIV therapies.

However, as discussed above, there may well be a role for IL-2 as an adjunct to vaccinations following depression of HIV levels and restoration of CD4$^+$ cell counts by triple or quadruple combination anti-viral therapies. In addition, given the theories on the skew away from T_h1 helper T-cell populations towards T_h2 as AIDS develops (Chapter 3), a role for IL-12 or IL-10 in reversing the skew back to T_h1 could be envisaged.

General.   Further developments in therapeutic viral vaccines will include the co-administration with immunomodulatory genes and proteins. Granulocyte colony stimulating factor (GMCSF) and other cytokines such as IL-12 have been used in animal models in order to boost and influence the immunological response to the antigen. Molecules such as these may be able to alter the global immune response around the antigen and stimulate T_h1 type responses (see Chapter 3) which theoretically should generate a stronger cell-mediated immunity. While several studies have shown promise in animal studies the principle remains to be demonstrated in the clinic. Nonetheless it is a promising technology which can be applied to both protein vaccines and naked DNA vaccines and developmental studies are ongoing.

References

1. Morse, S. (1996), *Emerging Viruses*. Oxford University Press, Oxford.

2. Vossen, R.C.R.M., Dam-Mieras, M.C.E. and Bruggeman, C.A. (1996) *Intervirology,* **39**, 213.
3. Corne, J.M. and Holgate, S.T. (1997) *Thorax,* **52**, 380.
4. Hegele, R.G. (1997) *Inf. Dis. Clin. Practice,* **6**, 167.
5. Davis-Poynter, N.J. and Farell, H. (1996) *Immunol. Cell Biol.,* **74**, 513.
6. Boursnell, M.E.G., Entwisle, D., Blakeley, D., Roberts, C., Duncan, I.A., Chisholm, S.E., Martin, G.M., Jennings, R., Challanian, D.N.I., Sobek, I., Inglis, S.C. and McLean, C.S. (1997) *J. Inf. Dis.,* **175**, 16.

Index

5-Fluorouracil, 129, 130, 132, 133

Accessory/auxiliary
  Vpr, 48
  Vpu, 48
  Vif, 49
Aciclovir
  antiviral activity, 5–6, 29, 31
  mechanism of action, 7–8, 31–32
  resistance, 33–34
  safety, 7
  triphosphate, 7, 31–33, 35–36
Acquired Immunodeficiency Syndrome
  (AIDS), 43
  dementias, 54
ADCC, 149
Adenosine arabinoside, 5, 6, 31
Adenoviruses, 72
Alzheimers Disease, 144
Amantadine hydrochloride, 16
  clinical studies, 79
  M2 ion channel, 78
  registered, 79
  resistance, 78
  structure, 78
  uncoating, 77
Animal models, 121, 134
Anti-sense, 132, 133
  ISIS, 29, 22, 35, 38
Apoptosis,
  cell cycle, 49
Arenavirus, 141
Assembly, 23
Attachment
  C3d, 22
  heparin sulphate, 22
  binding, 49

BDCRB, 35, 38
Bichloroacetic acid, 129
Borna virus, 145
  CD8+ T-cells, 145
Bovine papillomavirus – (BPV), 121–124,
  134–136
BVdU, 11, 35, 36

Caliciviridae, 98, 99

Canine oral papillomavirus (COPV),
  121, 136.
Cervical cancer, 124–128.
Chain termination
  AZT, 54, 144
  aciclovir, 31–33
  ganciclovir, 36
  penciclovir, 36
Chemokine receptors, 154
  CCKR5, 44, 49
  CXCR4, 44, 49
  CCR2, 154
  CCR3, 154
Chemokines
  AOP RANTES, 44, 154
  MetRANTES, 44, 154
  MIP1α, 44, 49
  MIP1β, 44, 49
  RANTES, 44, 49, 153
Chickenpox (see varicella zoster virus)
Chimpanzee, 102, 103, 118
Chronic acute hepatitis, 100, 105, 116
Cidofovir, 132, 133
Cirrhosis, 100, 105, 116
CMV retinitis, 43
CNS, 27, 30, 142
  canine distemper, 142
  EBV, 143
  HCMV, 143
  herpes, 142
  JC virus, 143
  measles, 142
  paramyxoviruses, 142
  poliovirus, 143
  retroviruses, 143
  rubella, 144
CO_2 laser, 130, 131
Cold sores, 24–26
Combination, 67–69, 140
  triple, 68
  quadruple, 68
  synergy, 68
Complement inactivation (retrovirus), 142
Coronaviruses, 72
Cottontail rabbit papillomavirus (CRPV),
  121, 135–136
Crystallisation, 56, 59–61
Cytokines, 133, 135
  IFNa, 44, 153
  IFNg, 44, 153
  IL-2, 44, 67

157